THE
CACTUS
SURGEON

Using Nature to Fix A Faulty Brain

Hannah Powell

Perrywood
Press

Published in 2021 by Perrywood Press

ISBN Paperback: 978-1-7399339-0-6
Ebook: 978-1-7399339-1-3

A CIP catalogue copy of this book can be found in the British Library.

Published with the help of Indie Authors World
www.indieauthorsworld.com

IndieAuthors
World

If you want to get better, or wish your body and mind would let you do more, this book is for you.

Acknowledgements

I started writing during a 2020 Covid-19 lockdown after signing up for the Michael Heppell Write That Book Masterclass. To Michael and my fellow authors, your support, guidance, chapter reviews, and good humour helped me get this over the line. Not perfect, but done!

I feel fortunate to have such a wonderful family. Mum and Dad, thank you for giving me many unique opportunities and for always believing in me. Simon and Tristan, thank you for your friendship, guidance and challenge. I'm proud to be your big sister. D and E, our journey has only just begun, and I look forward to many more adventures. Thank you, D, for being so kind and supportive every day, especially when I was ill. To my special E, you bring a smile to my face every day!

To my extended family, friends and the Perrywood team, who have been there for me through the ups and downs of life and shared my passions and interests along the way – thank you. Many people and events are not part of this memoir, but that doesn't mean they aren't important. There have been countless kindnesses and friendships bestowed on me over the years, for which I am eternally grateful.

These are my recollections and may not match the memories of others.

To my copy editor, Deborah Shaw, thank you for your brilliant suggestions, technical advice and encouragement. Jenny Williams, you are very wise and did a fantastic job of proofreading the final manuscript. To Rachel Kenny, who reviewed my first 10,000 words, your sage advice sat in my head as the words flowed. All three of you helped me improve my writing and find my voice. Kim and the team at Indie Authors World have cleverly guided me through the publishing process. Any mistakes are my own.

Finally, thank you to everyone who has been in touch to comment on my Cactus Surgeon social media posts and my e-book. I hoped my writing would help others, and this was my motivation to publish. Your positive comments kept me going and told me I was on the right track.

Prologue

I lay flat on my back, about to enter the tunnel. 'I need you to lie still for me, please, love,' said the kind technician. I tensed up and fought back the tears. If I could keep still, I wouldn't be here, worrying. As a distraction, I thought about the giant plane trees I went past to get here, trunks smooth yet mottled with greens and greys, thousands of leaves filtering London's dirty air. Luck was on my side, and, for once, my torso and limbs behaved themselves as the MRI machine whirred and clicked and juddered around me. I had never felt so terrified.

It all started in 2008. As I lay in bed, going to sleep, my body softly woke me with small movements, hardly noticeable, and I didn't think anything of it. But they increased and got to the point where they couldn't be ignored. I began to spasm in the daytime, generally while trying to relax, and it became more and more frequent. My physiotherapist was concerned and wrote a letter to my GP. Months later, I was in an MRI machine on the back of a lorry outside a hospital.

By then, I had a right hand tremor and twitched all the time with shoulder shrugs and forward movement in my torso, reacting to loud noises and touch. I rode a rollercoaster towards my diagnosis, and, as a result, my symptoms became more severe. At their worst, they were triggered when walking, hearing loud noises like fireworks, or picking up a piece of paper. I convulsed and threw my arms out in response. I looked like a peculiar air drummer with no rhythm. I came home from work on the Tube, my whole body jerking around uncontrollably. One caring soul noticed and gave up her seat. Everyone else just looked away. I got off at the station and perched on a roadside bollard, rain and tears mixing as they poured down my face.

These problems with my nervous system changed my life. For a month I didn't often leave our South London flat. I didn't return to work for six months and have never gone back full-time. With not much information to help me, and in striving for better health, I found ways to keep the symptoms, anxiety and stress at bay and want to share my experiences with you.

To move forward, I've had to look back and reflect. I'm sharing my personal journey, hoping that it will inspire you to make positive changes or understand other people a little bit better. I'll outline how I overcame depression and burnout, and how I celebrate the small wonders of nature which continue to keep me grounded.

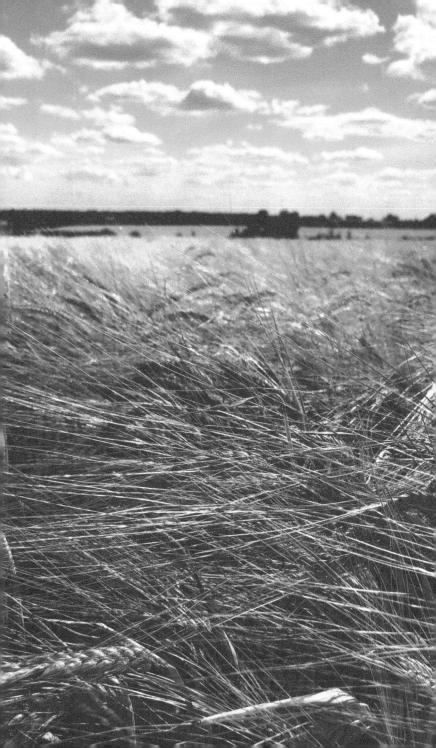

Chapter 1

In hindsight, my sudden period of lousy health started years earlier. I moved to London in the early noughties, after university, and threw myself into both work and play. I had jobs where I would regularly graft from 8 a.m. to 8 p.m., after which we would either pile down the pub or collapse in exhaustion in front of the TV. Self-care was not on the agenda.

I trudged through a series of temporary jobs: staffing reception on the twenty-sixth floor of Canary Wharf, stuffing envelopes for Holborn lawyers and doing my best to get closer to something related to my horticulture degree. In contrast to my green upbringing, I came home after work to a modern townhouse near the northern end of the Blackwall Tunnel. To get there I walked past the Robin Hood Gardens estate, built in the 1960s and designed to look like 'streets in the sky'. In reality, they were grey, depressing and noisy (at least from the outside; I've never been in), and intimidating after dark. One November, we had to watch out for fireworks being thrown at us and we walked quickly past like alert soldiers on patrol.

Despite this grey backdrop and the uncertainty of unemployment, life was a fun extension of my student days.

I held onto bright moments, like our small patch of lawn bathed in sunlight before the shadows of tall buildings snatched it away. Or catching the briefest glimpse of blue on a magpie's wing whilst commuting at the front of a Docklands Light Railway carriage. I escaped home to Essex when it all got too much. The optimism of youth kept me plugging away, determined to plough my own furrow and carve out a compelling career.

My temping finally paid off and landed me a role with a top West End PR agency. I would be within touching distance of the BBC Radio 1 studios, the iconic BT Tower and the oh-so-cool Charlotte Street bars and restaurants.

I'd left behind a childhood where I'd grown up working for and intertwined with my parents' garden centre. Luck and dogged persistence found me a workplace with a similar family feel. They took a rough-round-the-edges girl from rural Essex under their wing and taught me more than I could have imagined.

As a teenager, I read Downtown, by Anne Rivers Siddons, about a rural girl entering life as a writer in the big city of Atlanta. I desperately wanted the camaraderie, the high jinks and the sense of belonging that Smoky O'Donnell immersed herself in – and at the PR agency I'd finally found it, in spades.

For the first few months, I earned respect and proved my worth, assisting my team, taking on extra jobs and asking, all the time, when can I be promoted? Finally, after a year, I got my wish. I started attending client meetings and taking their calls. Taking deep breaths, I picked up the phone to cold call journalists – which, like Marmite, I absolutely hated. My love affair with writing began. I often edited press releases amongst clouds of other people's smoke on late evenings, glass of wine in hand. My boss sometimes drank too much, so we'd water down her wine when she wasn't looking. Ignoring her request to press send, we'd save her drunken ramblings for revision in the cold light of the next day. We should have gone home hours earlier.

I was young, worry-free on the surface and having a ball. I could always find someone to go to the pub with on any night of the week. On Fridays, we'd gather in the breakout area. We'd clap at the week's successes, eat insubstantial nibbles and drink copious amounts of free wine and beer – before stumbling to a nearby pub to carry on into the night.

I said I would run around the office (all three floors) in just my bra and jeans if we raised enough money for charity. Even my bemused parents chipped in, and we exceeded the required target. In the toilets, I nervously swapped my own bra for a somewhat larger double D scarlet version. I'd bought it especially for the occasion, and my trembling fingers stuffed the extra space full of tissue paper. If I was going to do this – and it was way too late to back out now – I might as well put on a show. I shook all over like a terrified dog and would have whimpered too if I'd been able to find my voice. Taking a deep breath, I pulled open the door to make a mad dash for it. I didn't hang around. Everyone had gathered to whoop and cheer as I rushed by, my head down, trying to look bright and breezy. Back in the toilets, the shaking finally disappeared, and I looked into the mirror, smiling. Even ill-judged comments about me 'blushing all over' couldn't take away from the fact that I'd entered office folklore. I'd also raised £500 for charity.

Deskbound near a window, I could see only the bricks and tiles of other tall buildings. I craved green - anything to break up the grey. As the days started to lengthen, I left in the light, surprised and blinking like a mole emerging from its tunnel. One evening, without even thinking about it, I extended my journey to pass through Fitzroy Square. Its private garden behind black metal railings equally intrigued and frustrated me; I shook the lock to find it shut fast. Defeated, I descended into the dark depths of the Northern line. When I popped up again, the light had gone for another day.

In May of my first year in London, I went to the famous Kew Gardens with a date. Just being there made my heart sing; I loved being surrounded by trees from around the world and, as we walked round hand in hand, I liked to test my knowledge. When I got the plant name before I looked at the name tag, I was triumphant. I kept up a running botany-based commentary. It's a habit inherited from my dad, and thankfully my suitor found it endearing rather than annoying.

Colleagues occasionally wheeled me out for my horticultural prowess, such as when we pitched for the business of the Apple and Pear Development Council. We travelled to the meeting by Tube, train and taxi, holding a colossal apple and pear pie with flaky, golden pastry fruits on top. I proudly recited my BSc Horticulture 2:1 qualification during our nervous introductions. Sadly, even the finest baked goods and a relevant degree were not enough to win their business.

Our routine of monthly client meetings rolled around soon enough, including north of the Capital, in Milton Keynes. We travelled by train, at first discussing how we would present our reports, before chatting or making the most of an opportunity to chill out. Once we left the suburbs and got into the countryside the yellow fields drew my eyes.

It was high summer and the sight of a combine, a soaring red kite or a field full of black-and-white cows gave me a quick thrill. I kept these thoughts to myself, wondering if anyone else in the carriage had also spotted them, smiling to think they might be there for me alone. Alighting in Milton Keynes, my mind switched back to work and we caught a cab to the Domino's Pizza offices. It was a lunchtime meeting and, yes, pizza was on the menu. On the way home we had to stand swaying on the jam-packed train. Purposely near the door for the view, I let the train rock me into a trance as the fields once again whizzed past. I realised how tired I was.

Financial journalists from the Sunday papers sometimes rang me on a Friday night. I would invariably be in a noisy pub, and I'd fight through the crowds and a gentle tipsiness to stand nervously on the pavement outside and repeat the party line. After the final call, I could switch off my phone, let the tension depart and knock back the wine.

Me and most of my colleagues were 'always on', with little or no regard for work-life balance. Working at full throttle would later take its toll, and external events would test my resilience.

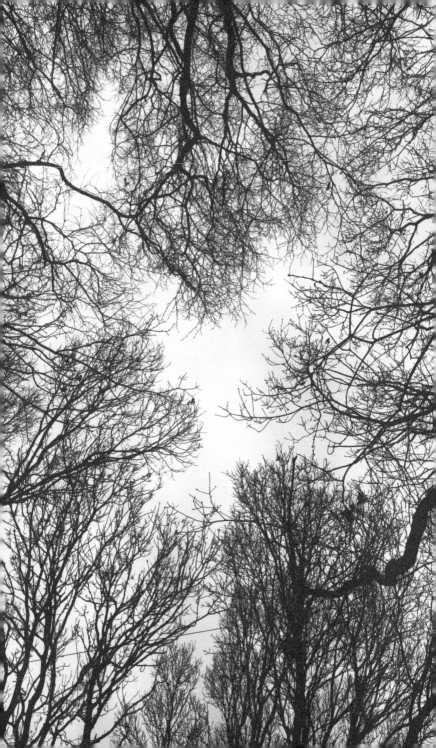

Chapter 2

I had never been to a funeral until 2001. That year, I attended several. We lost my grandad and my aunt's mum, an extra grandmother in all but name. Harder to reconcile was Dad's best man tragically dying after falling off a ladder. I could suddenly see my own parents' mortality in front of me.

But Mat's death hit me like a juggernaut.

I knew I wouldn't see him again because Mum and Dad had already been to say goodbye to him at the hospice. The night before, I'd had the call to say he had gone, and I went to work the next day thinking I had no more tears to cry. Standing at the photocopier, hurt and pain bubbled up and I wiped my wet cheeks as I realised I would grow older than him. He is forever young, stuck at twenty-six.

The previous week had seen more than 2,000 people killed in the Twin Towers attack. The world was focused on that devastating loss, whilst my world had been ripped apart much closer to home. Death followed me around, especially on the Tube. Strangers stood over me, and headlines fell from their newspaper pages into my peripheral vision. Snatches of conversations between friends or colleagues whirled around me. We all tried to make sense of these tragic events.

I'd never before met another young person who liked plants as much as I did. I'd worked alongside Mat in our plant nursery, and he absolutely loved growing. He had a true passion for acers - trees and shrubs dramatic in spring when the leaves unfurl to reveal bright and vivid colours, or in autumn when they put on an equally impressive show before falling to the ground. Before that, I felt like I belonged in an adult world, old before my time. There were two versions of Hannah: the one where I lived and breathed plants, then another at school and with my friends, just another acne-afflicted teen desperate to fit in. Loving plants didn't help with this at all.

The day of his funeral came, and we all got in the car, trying to hold it together for each other. We were on show, Mum and Dad being his employers as well as his friends. They wanted to hold back the emotion for as long as they could. My carefully constructed dam broke, and I scrabbled in my bag for a wad of tissues. I tried not to catch anyone's eye. Silent in our grief, nothing could be said to bring comfort.

We shuffled into a packed church, as befitted his popularity. Then followed the last chance to say goodbye. As the coffin disappeared into the ground, Dad stepped forward and, in tears, threw a branch of one of Mat's acers on top. A tender gesture that broke my heart.

A cloak of grief descended. It was impossible to shake it off. When the phone rang, my heart beat harder. Had something else bad happened? Kind friends took me for strolls around the block, or invited me to stay at theirs after a night out, when they could see that life had become too much for me. Small gestures had a big impact. I took a week off work to get myself together.

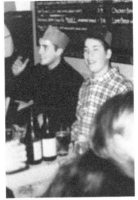

Mat and Simon

I was unsure about going for counselling, but I knew something needed to change. I enjoyed walking to my counsellor's North London house past front gardens packed full of soothing trees and shrubs. I could see vivid colours through the railings, hear the wind caressing their stems and even stroked trunks and furry leaves as they bent over the walls to distract me.

Springtime is the most glorious season and boosts my spirits no end. I passed flowering magnolias – both the subtle star-shaped stellata and the bigger, blowsier grandiflora strutting their stuff. Branches of catkins drooped over walls and puffed out their pollen in the breeze. My eyes watered with hay fever, but it's worth suffering for spring. Pink and white cherry blossom burst out into blue skies with abandon. Noticing natural changes on the way to each visit eased me into the sessions. I started by commenting on my observations. It somehow grounded me when I most needed it.

I am strongly connected to the seasons, preferring the buzz and potential of spring to the flatness of winter. The darker months are always when it's hardest to shake off a cloak of sadness. When the sap rises in the trees in spring, my energy typically returns, at least for a while.

**

Four years later, my mental health had improved and I'd been promoted twice more at work. On the day of the 7/7 bombings, I had a doctor's appointment, so didn't get on the Northern line as I usually would. Later, I arrived to find the station shut, following an incident. I went home and switched on the TV to discover that many people had been killed in Tube carriages and on a bus. Minutes felt like hours, and hours dragged out interminably as I sat there alone, worrying about everyone I knew. My friends and colleagues didn't die, but still, London was a bad dream. Mayor Ken Livingstone told the world we were resilient but I was just tired and lonely. I stepped reluctantly onto the tube each morning and evening. I had to use public transport. I didn't have a choice.

Despite the threats of city living, I didn't always act sensibly. One evening, after a boozy Christmas lunch and an afternoon of drinking, we bundled a drunk colleague into a taxi we hailed off the street and waved her goodbye. In our glee that we'd found her a ride, we didn't realise that it wasn't a black cab. She woke up in the taxi to find it parked up and the driver in the back with her. She managed to get away before he did anything. Still, I felt terrible and very guilty about the part I played in this incident.

Despite being surrounded by the largest group of friends I had ever had, an underlying sadness shrouded me. Is this why I couldn't stop drinking on a night out? I didn't have an off switch. Being alone with my thoughts could be overwhelming. I stayed out late until the alcohol sent them to sleep.

Externally living my best life, I ignored signs that, inside, my mind and body were struggling, driving me towards disaster. What's more, my drinking put me in some embarrassing situations.

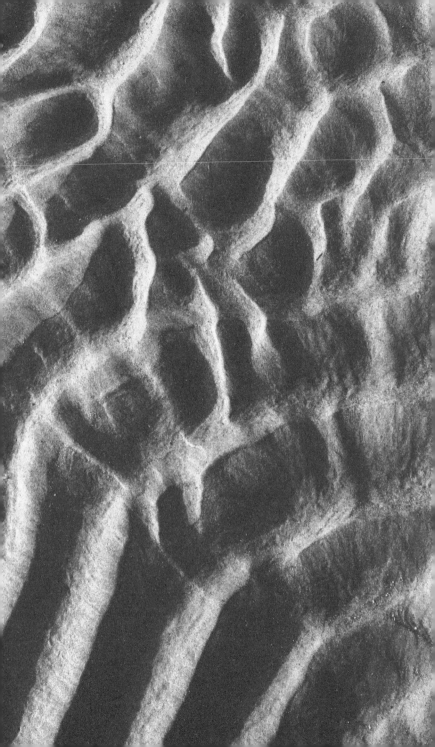

Chapter 3

At the start of the evening, I looked terrific in my figure-hugging silk combat trousers and tight, bright pink top. Hours later, tummy full of cava and wine and dressed as the singer Pink, I kissed a cowboy on the dance floor in front of all my colleagues. I caught glimpses of my bright cerise lipstick smeared across his face.

I woke alone in my bed the following morning and the events of the night before hit me right between the eyes. A horrible movie played on repeat in my head. What on earth did I do that for? Head throbbing, I picked up my trademark hangover sausage sandwich – brown toast, brown sauce – to delay the office walk of shame.

Sitting at my desk, the bright lipstick might have been gone, but the evening had left a stain on my character. Having been seen stuck together like glue, the cowboy and I now studiously ignored each other. We sat and wallowed in our shared embarrassment across the inconveniently open-plan office. A week later, he came out to his colleagues, and my shame boiled over again.

Our client Barclaycard's sponsorship of the Premier League took me into the previously unknown world of football. We held glitzy, glam launch parties in Manchester and London. We invited players and coaches from all twenty teams, and I looked at hundreds of pictures of young female models so we could pay them to come along in football kits and Reebok Classic trainers. I managed to mumble some words when I greeted the legendary Alex Ferguson but had no idea who the confident man with a short fat tie was. He strode up to our desk of name badges and said, 'Dean Holdsworth, plus one.' A colleague took over; thankfully she recognised Dean's plus one as Bolton manager and future England manager Sam Allardyce. At the after-parties, the drinks flowed as we celebrated a great event. I bathed in the day's successes, and never had an empty glass. Sat next to the Barclaycard CEO, I touched his knee whilst leaning in a bit close to tell a joke. To my surprise, the next day, and for several weeks, colleagues teased me for sitting on his knee. I don't think I did, but we had consumed an awful lot of champagne.

The impressive hangar-like Tate Modern turbine hall was the venue for an online gaming launch hosted by Ant and Dec. The TV stars had earned their exorbitant fee and gone, so we took the after-party upstairs, drinking yet more cava, with only a few micro canapés in our still-rumbling tummies. I weaved my way towards a client I had never spoken to before. The room spun, but he held me up as we kissed urgently in the corner.

As the event came to a close, I needed to find a taxi. The object of my affection had scarpered, and we never did have a conversation. My senior client – oh no, the person I was supposed to impress – offered to drop me off in his cab. We headed south and he took fatherly responsibility for me. I got in and immediately fell into a deep sleep, head occasionally jerking upwards as I roused momentarily. Later, he shook me awake and asked me exactly where I lived.

'Balham High Street,' I mumbled, 'above Iceland.'

I'd swapped East London for South, still living next to a busy thoroughfare. The taxi waited while I got my key in the lock. It took an eternity. I attempted a wave and stumbled upstairs straight into bed. I discarded clothes where they fell. I woke the next morning with a pounding headache and a sick, shameful feeling in my stomach. It hit me hard: a sense that I'd lost control of my faculties and couldn't prevent the story from being played out. Yet again, a non-existent film reel stuck on repeat.

Flamboyant Christmas party venues included a golf hotel, a drag club, an Italian restaurant and a lunch in Paris. Regrettably, I have no memory of the beautiful French city save for some lovely red velvet curtains and being poured more wine during our déjeuner. We had a carriage to ourselves on the Eurostar, which resulted in further heavy drinking on the return journey. Carnage. For once, some of the others were snogging with hands all over each other in front of absolutely everyone. At Waterloo, we disembarked, and a few of us literally fell into another bar.

At Madame Jojo's in Soho, with a headgear fancy dress theme, Ruth and I dressed as Playboy bunnies. Wearing short black skirts and large white-and-pink rabbit ears, we found it easier to enter the venue as a matching pair. A graduate gave someone (in a long-term relationship) a blow job in the broom cupboard. The queens on stage guffawed when they noticed a commotion and the couple emerged from the closet.

Another year, another party. Was it any surprise to be somewhat intoxicated by 10 p.m.? Our whole company had been transported by coach to a sophisticated golf hotel somewhere in the home counties, and some of us were about to disgrace ourselves. I came back from hitching up my baggy-round-the-crotch tights in the toilets, tottering in kitten heels, and weighed up who to hang out with next. A small yet exuberant group spotted me and dragged me into their sparkling orbit. I blindly followed them on their mission as they stumbled with purpose towards the hotel's bank of golf buggies. After the initial disappointment of no keys, Emma managed to hotwire one using her ring. I stood agog until someone pulled me onto a seat next to them. We were off! The driver tried to take us towards an A-road.

Coming from nowhere, a couple of security guards in high-vis coats loomed out of the darkness, and the light of their high-strength torch beams struck my face. I froze. Visions of every prison break movie I'd ever watched ran through my head. I am not a rule breaker and was immediately appalled at myself. A deep male voice hailed us with a megaphone, 'Stop, or we will call the police.'

The driver immediately stopped the buggy, and everyone bolted except for me. I stood up, lit up by their torchlight and apologised for our misdemeanour, wailing, 'I'm so sorry. I'm really very sorry.'

The others kindly returned to drag me away. Thankfully, the security guards seemed content to get their buggy back and, despite my worst fears, I made it back to the bar to do another round of shots. The next morning, I woke in my hotel room rather than a police cell.

At the hotels we stayed in, and in the bathrooms of the bars we visited, people disappeared to do coke; not interested myself I was vaguely aware it existed. One day, we had an anthrax scare when someone discovered white powder in the post room; we had some high-profile clients who could have been targeted. It wasn't anthrax ...

For years I beat myself up about drinking too much and was far too hard on myself. I have learned to see events for what they were – drunken events typical of a twenty-something PR person working in an industry which encouraged and normalised habitual drinking.

I had no idea about the dangers of drinking too much and the effect it can have on your body and mind. I drank to be more confident and to push away underlying feelings of sadness. I pushed them away, without realising they would bubble up again one day.

After many unlucky dates and relationships, and having moved three times in four years, something needed to change. It was time to put down some roots.

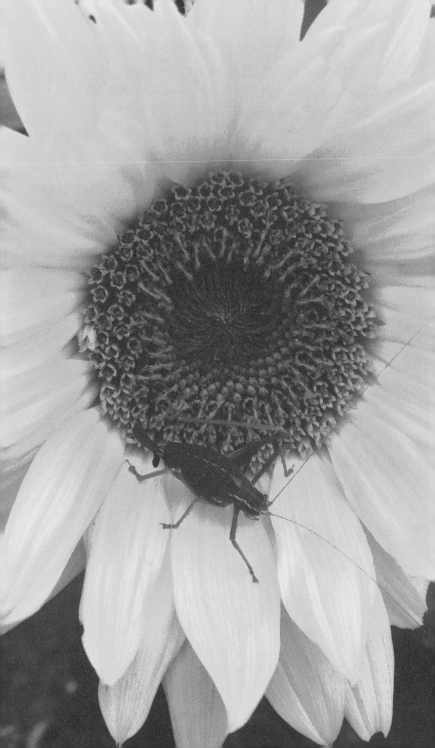

Chapter 4

I bought my first home: a first-floor maisonette with Victorian wooden sash windows and a sunshine yellow front door that made me smile as I entered. Concrete stairs from the kitchen led down to my first-ever garden, a handkerchief-sized patio with a raised brick flower bed. A skinny grey fox created her den there under a prickly berberis bush, making me too nervous to use the space whilst she reared her young. When I'd go out the back door, she'd leave her babies and jump away over the fence. I didn't want to meet an angry returning vixen. Instead, I sat on the top doorstep when the sun shone, a cup of Earl Grey in my hand, enjoying the view of trees and plants in other people's gardens.

One Saturday morning, I woke up jaded, hungover and uneasy. We'd gone out the previous night on Old Compton Street in Soho and the details blurred in my mind. I had no concrete plans for the rest of the weekend. The silence deafened me, so I wandered aimlessly from room to room and tried but failed to motivate myself out of my gloom.

I answered my phone to find Mum checking in on me. She gave me some tough maternal love and told me in no uncertain terms to go for a walk. Begrudgingly, I hung up and went out towards Tooting Common. At first, my tense shoulders hunched over whilst sadness and hopelessness circled like vultures round and round my head. Batting the feelings away didn't work. They persisted. I hated my inner voice. It didn't sound like me, yet it invaded my usual positive outlook, as I waded through treacle.

Slowly pounding the pavements, I began to unfurl like a fern in spring. Here and there in tiny front gardens I discovered splashes of colour - breaking up the identical doorsteps and over-filled dustbins. Admiring a pot of scarlet tulips, I was ten years old again, coming face-to-face with pollen-laden bees as they shot out of the black centres. Further along, the can't-be-missed yellow of fluffy pom-pom mimosa flowers shouted out, 'Look at me!' By the time I reached the park, the tension had gone, and I stretched my arms out like a cat lying in the sunshine.

I ambled with no route in mind. Being surrounded by strangers, each with their own private thoughts and reasons for being there, comforted me. Signs of emerging life sprang out everywhere. A red admiral butterfly landed on a leaf, showing off its brown wings with orange and white spots. At the pond, I stopped and sat on a bench, and watched the swans and moorhens. An elderly lady passed, wrapped up in her winter coat, hat and gloves in the weak spring sunshine. She smiled at me, enjoying the scene. I beamed back, appreciating this unexpected connection, and pushed myself up, ready to go.

In the flat, I made a cup of tea, humming to myself. The walk had shifted and lifted my mood. I suddenly became aware that my black thoughts had gone, at least for the moment. With renewed vigour and a sense of purpose, I visited the supermarket to pick up groceries. A bunch of tulips also went into the shopping basket. They would sit in a striped vase on my wooden kitchen table to remind me of happier times.

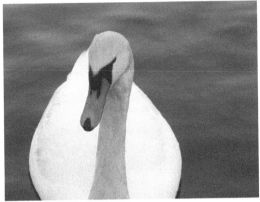

Serene swan

I cherished my holidays. They provided an escape from urban surroundings, from my flummoxed frustration that I remained single whilst friends coupled up and got married. I'd had some great trips to the hotter climes of southern Europe but it wasn't always easy to find someone to go on holiday with, so next time I went solo.

After a long transatlantic flight to San José, Costa Rica, I found my ride and we headed towards the hotel. Looking out of the window, I saw tall fences and barbed wire surrounding every house and building. I didn't feel welcome, and the butterflies in my stomach were turning into rocks.

Briefed on arrival, we were warned not to leave the hotel alone and not to go out in the dark. What had I got myself into? After a deep breath into the bathroom mirror, I left to meet the other travellers, coming across friendly smiles and an easy-going teacher roommate. The next day, as we left the capital behind for the countryside, the barbed wire fences and my nerves faded away. Our chatter became less stilted with each hour, and we started to build and test fragile alliances.

Everything was new to my wide eyes. Fields whizzed by full of lush green coffee bushes or low, spiky pineapples – as far as the eye could see. We stopped at a roadside stall to eat wedges of the fresh fruit, juice dripping down our chins, and drink fresh coconut water. My taste buds had never felt so alive.

At night, we discovered tarantulas by shining our torches into holes in tree trunks. Warned not to touch anything in the humid cloud forest of Monteverde, we didn't need to be told twice. The air hummed with chirping, ribbiting and grunting, scores of frogs trying to attract a mate.

At another roadside stop, we saw a sloth, algae and lichen on its fur, hanging in a tree. I have never been a fan of long nails, perhaps because the dirt got into mine and stained them whilst gardening, so I am fastidious about keeping them regularly trimmed. In comparison, the sloth had the longest, most revolting nails I had ever seen, although they are actually sharp claws, strong enough to keep them in the trees. Endearing facial markings made it look like it was smiling and I forgot the nails as I fell in love with this bizarre creature which did everything at one speed – slow.

Tour guide Bernie had sharp eyes and pointed out flora and fauna. Once I got my eye in, I soon spotted toucans and the colourful quetzal, reminding me of Roald Dahl's Roly-Poly Bird. Many of the plants were familiar to my eyes but resided indoors in the UK. We visited a homestead in the hills; in Annie's garden, we came across an eight-foot-high poinsettia looking lush and resplendent, even though it was months away from Christmas. I couldn't believe the number of Bromeliads, brightly coloured spiky-leafed plants which grow on trees, collecting water in their rosette centres, and was taken aback to find there are more than 2,000 species in Costa Rica. Likewise, I found out that there are 1,300 species of Orchid, some of which are pollinated by hummingbirds. Everywhere we went, my eyes popped out on stalks. There was an abundance of super-sized plants and animals.

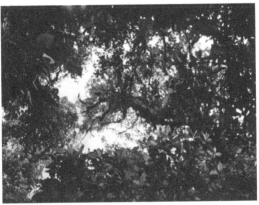

Looking up into the tree canopy

On the beach of Tortuguero one night, we crept in small groups to see a most wondrous sight. In front of us sat a loggerhead turtle, a huge, lumbering creature, depositing soft, ping-pong ball eggs into an enormous hole in the sand. We sat bathed in moonlight using additional UV lamps to watch unseen as she did her duty. She used her flippers to cover the eggs, and we winced to see how little sand she could move with each clumsy movement – like a human filling a sandpit one teaspoon at a time. It must have taken her ages to dig the hole. She remained focused on the task at hand. Eventually, job done, she propelled herself down the beach and into the sea. For a moment, her clumsiness turned into grace. Then she disappeared under the waves. She gave no fond farewells, or backward looks. I wondered what it must be like to never see your babies. For those minutes, immersed in her world, mine paled into insignificance.

Being close to nature in such a profound way was incredibly moving. I departed for home with some much-needed perspective and more energy.

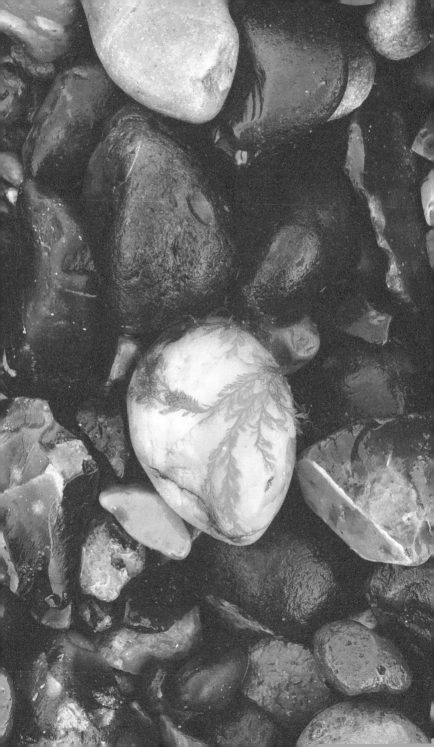

Chapter 5

After five years in PR, I left and took on a role promoting entrepreneurship from a draughty industrial-style office in Covent Garden. On my first day, I emerged from a bustling Waterloo Station and walked north across Golden Jubilee Bridge. My stomach whirled unpredictably like the seagulls above me, but my breath slowed at the sight of the Thames. Its brown beguiling waters held my attention until a fast-paced trainer-wearing commuter jostled me for being in the way. Crossing the bridge became my daily meditation. Even soaked to the bone, high on adrenaline or running on empty, the river soothed me and filled my thoughts.

In my new job, I became a campaigner striving for change. I travelled to Budapest, Paris and Washington DC to discuss and run masterclasses on promoting entrepreneurship. Invited to the British Ambassador residences in Paris and Budapest, we listened to the ambassador speak in his garden of mature trees whilst the sun went down behind us. In Washington, I added on a couple of days to make the most of my first visit to this historic city – marvelling equally at how modest the White House seemed and how large the watermelon radishes and heirloom tomatoes looked at the farmers' market.

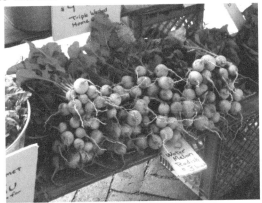

Watermelon radish

Working with others to run the annual Global Entrepreneurship Week was incredible yet intense. Again, we worked hard, often typing away late into the night when other offices had long gone home. Our challenge was to galvanise many countries and thousands of UK schools, colleges, businesses and community organisations to run events in the same week. Together we could encourage young people to set up their own businesses.

Nights out continued, still on the agenda. In Liverpool for our Christmas party, we found ourselves in a deserted underground club and took over the dance floor. I have always loved dancing (with no particular skill or grace) and attempted to launch myself up into the air off my boss's shoulders. As I pushed myself off, sharp, severe pain stopped me in my tracks. I'd partially dislocated my shoulder, but luckily it popped back in straight away. I had never sobered up so quickly and, for me, the night had ended. Coming home on the train the next day, I sat pale and grey faced, my arm hanging limply, not even able to delight in the countryside scenes we flashed past.

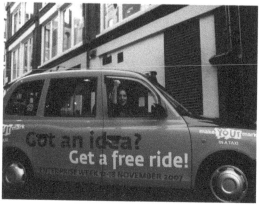

Taxi!

In this job, I engaged in discussions about politics for the first time. I discovered that, unlike in North Essex, blue was not the only colour. Working for a campaigning organisation partly funded by government, I encountered politicians and civil servants and, whilst some of them were lovely, others simply frustrated me.

Peter Mandelson, MP and business minister, asked us to produce a video (with him in) for National Enterprise Day, to play in every school in the country. Not particularly inspiring for young people. Oh, and he gave us just four weeks. Thanks, Peter, for another stress-inducing period of late nights. I became familiar with the vanity and short-term outlook of those in power. We attended monthly meetings in the Department for Business, which always gave me a headache. Just being in that building was energy sapping, not least because we were never offered a drink.

While work cracked on at a pace, my dating attempts stuttered and floundered, until I met D. Unlike the others, I didn't need to try and like him. Chaperoned by our mutual friend James on our first date, we sat in the Princess Louise pub in Holborn, me laughing at the two of them. Amateur comics with a university radio show and podcast under their belts, they amused me with their natural double act. Our first dates took place in London's many pubs and restaurants, our first kiss on Waterloo Bridge overlooking the river. We escaped to Cornwall for our first weekend away, and spent many hours on the coastal paths. We discovered a mutual love for hiking and being outdoors. This, despite him only ever having lived in Birmingham and London. A man who found me attractive in fleece-lined walking trousers was a keeper. That, and he cleaned my oven the first time he visited my flat.

At work, the hard graft continued. The BBC offered us access to the high-profile dragons from Dragons' Den and The Apprentice star Alan Sugar. Brilliant, but oh no, just two weeks' notice. Just a venue, 100 schoolchildren and marketing materials to be found. More late nights required.

At 6 p.m. one evening a few weeks after my birthday, my fingers flew over the keyboard, as I rushed to finish before going for a very expensive massage. Thoughtfully gifted to me by D, the scented oils called me. I called the hotel spa to see if I could move the 7 p.m. appointment, but it was impossible at such short notice. I had a difficult decision to make. Did I let my boss down or let D down by wasting his money? Either way, I lost out. The 7 p.m. appointment came and went as I remained focused on my task, angry and chained to my desk.

My eyes boggled as I passed through the famous black door of 10 Downing Street, which swung silently open as we approached. After taking our mobiles, a man in a grey suit invited us to go up the stairs past the recognisable bright yellow walls filled with black-and-white pictures of past prime ministers. I tried to look nonchalant and keep my mouth from falling open. The impressive reception room had high, white walls covered in decorative plasterwork. Just in front of me, a man tripped on a camera cable and fell towards me. Instinctively, I put my arms out to catch him, but luckily he righted himself without my assistance. This time my mouth did hang open as MP Neil Kinnock smiled at me sheepishly.

Another year, another Global Entrepreneurship Week, this time in a building swept for bombs by the security detail. Our event was running late, and we nervously kept the next high-profile speaker waiting in a small kitchen until he could be let out on stage. Prime Minister Gordon Brown took it all in his stride and spoke eloquently and passionately about education and entrepreneurship in his soft Scottish accent.

As an antidote to city life, and as the tarmac and concrete started to drag me down, I again subconsciously sought out plants and nature. I took the longer route from the Tube station to go past pocket-size parks and squares full of trees and mown green grass rather than the shorter routes that held no appeal. I observed minor changes as the seasons passed. Yellow leaves fell silently to the pavement. A late frost hung onto seed heads and parakeets demanded to be heard above the traffic.

On the train home to Essex at weekends, my shoulders softened and moved away from my ears. We'd chug away from graffitied walls and urban sprawl into flat, familiar fields. I strode the boundaries of the twelve-acre garden centre and adjoining woodland, with a need to check everything and reconnect. I passed the dead oak tree, once destroyed by lightning, catching fire whilst we slept in our beds. In the morning, we'd found its bark on the field twenty metres away, thrown aside by the powerful force of nature and an explosion of hot sap. Its silhouette was part of the landscape I knew so well. Like the back of my hand, it has changed as we've grown older, but it's always mine.

I'd prowl up and down the nursery greenhouses and say hello to those in the team I still recognised. To newer team members, I was a stranger in my own territory. Around the kitchen table, we'd fall into old habits, discussing the latest building projects, talking about the weather and blooming flowers. When I returned to London, I left part of me behind in Essex.

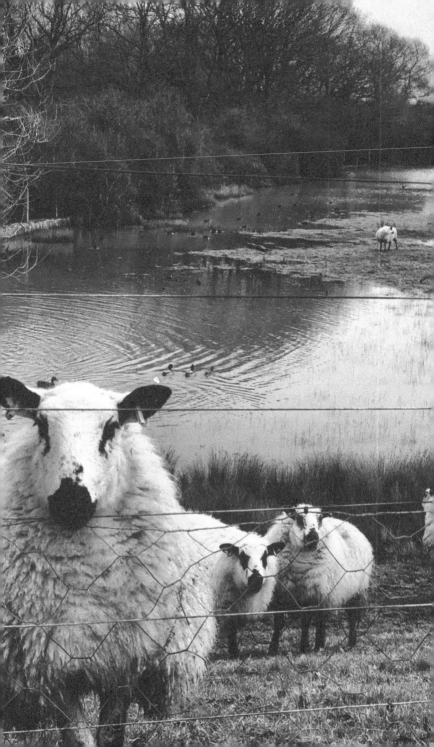

Chapter 6

The twitches began while I was in this job and going out with D. As I lay in bed going to sleep, my body softly woke me with minor movements, hardly noticeable. I didn't think anything of it. But they increased and got to the point where they could not be ignored.

I set off on a journey of discovery but first one of uncertainty. Google showed me my possible futures, and I did not like what might come to pass. The weeks and months dragged past, and I still didn't have a verdict. The stress of never-ending tests, appointments and endless worrying was not good for me. My symptoms got worse. Work signed me off for a couple of weeks, then more; I eventually took six months off to recover and get my life back on track.

At every appointment, a different expert bandied about yet another possible prognosis. I hung onto every word. I looked up the terms they mentioned as soon as I could. I grasped at any straw and clung on to any possible hope of finding what was wrong because it might lead to treatment and an end to this nightmare. I wanted an explanation and needed to explain to people what was happening to me.

In an appointment before the MRI scan, the consultant told me I had epilepsy – and prescribed medication that made no difference. At a later appointment, he informed me I probably had a condition called propriospinal myoclonus: irritation on the spine due to infection or a virus. He prescribed clonazepam to help control the muscle twitches. This also made no difference. Both theories were eventually disproven.

I mistakenly sent an email to work, family and friends telling them I had propriospinal myoclonus and informed them that it is relatively rare – the neurologist had never seen a case before. This update turned out to be premature and completely wrong.

The whole experience wore me out and I felt like it would never end. Some days I slept all day, others I wept until the rivers ran dry. Up to this point, I'd had little experience of coping with illness. I had had glandular fever as a student. I'd napped a lot, but most students do that anyway, and I had friends to keep me company, so it didn't seem too bad. I'd also tackled overwhelming depression, but those around me told me with conviction that I would get through it – and I did.

After they ruled out propriospinal myoclonus, the consultant invited four colleagues into the room to look at my symptoms because they did not fit their typical list. He asked me to put on a somewhat surreal show. Luckily, like a circus elephant, I performed on cue, and they witnessed the jerky back and arm movements. Their medical discussion passed me by, but the friendly head of the clinic assured me that they could sort me out. So, I just needed to wait for the next round of tests.

Each day, I only committed to getting out for a walk around the docks and the river where I'd moved to live with D. Even on the days when I couldn't go far, I went to the water to see the horizon and remind myself of the world at large. I set myself the challenge of taking one good photo every day. Some were of manufactured objects – textured rope on the dock, architecture, or street photography of people sitting on benches.

More life-affirming were the small wonders of nature. I became fanatical about them, and they gave me a reason to get dressed and go out. This was no mean feat, as walking triggered my twitches. Many of the photos featured plants, mosses and lichen. I came across details that others would stride past in their haste to get somewhere. A heart-shaped crevice in a pavement that someone had filled with bright yellow dandelions. A large-bodied brown spider, sitting in its web, waiting for dinner to land. A coot building a sad nest of discarded rubbish: plastic, string and crisp packets. While I looked and closely observed, all other thoughts disappeared, and the clouds lifted to leave me with a chink of hope.

I saw hanging purple wisteria immersed in the spring sunshine, swathes of pink campion flowers in luxuriant green grass alongside the pavement, swans and grebes nesting, and pots full of herbs and vegetables on houseboats. On days when I couldn't leave the flat, I took pictures of our houseplants or sat gazing at the London plane trees filling our window with a hundred shades of green. My life was in limbo but, around me, I saw plants growing, seasons changing, and I unearthed moments of pure joy. Seeking out these positives played a considerable part in helping me heal. I sensed that, without a break from thinking about being ill

Hannah Powell

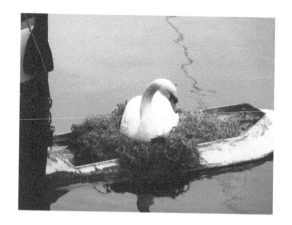

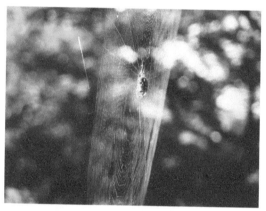

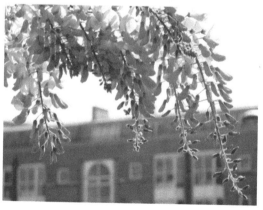

and feeling wretched, my body and brain wouldn't be able to move on. It would forget how to be well and get stuck.

As I walked, the contact between foot and ground caused my brain to overreact, and my torso and limbs jerked and moved in response. After much searching, I found comfortable Merrell shoes with bouncy soles. In them, I didn't feel the pressure so much and the reactions lessened. With relief, and, not knowing how long this would go on for, I stockpiled two more pairs.

Next to a community garden, I spotted a sign that said, 'Our Marguerite (daisy) was stolen by some sad and evil person.' Then in small font underneath, 'May their roots wither and die.' That piece of humour made my day.

Twenty-four hours seemed like forever, so my regular walks became a much-needed diversion from my downward-spiralling thoughts. On good days, I kept going to reach the Thames. This area had a different atmosphere: busy and full of life, with the bustle of riverboats ferrying commuters, workers and shoppers across the water to Canary Wharf. I'd nearly come full circle. My first home in London could be found the same distance from this dramatic skyline but on the other side of the river.

Sometimes I went in the opposite direction towards Southwark Park, past the brick-terraced house with a blue plaque telling me that Michael Caine grew up there. In the park, parakeets squawked in the trees and groups of long-tailed tits flittered about. As I took in the scene, yet more birds kept appearing: tufted ducks, swans and geese.

I loved going to Stave Hill Ecological Park and Russia Dock Woodland when I had a little more oomph. There are over five acres of nature on the site of Stave Dock. The docks were filled with rubble and waste from all over the capital after becoming derelict in the '70s. Landscapers used some of that rubble to construct the park and build a viewing platform on Stave Hill. Before the dock was built, it would have been pasture and, before that, a woodland wilderness. It's lovely to think it has gone full circle. Here, the flash of a turquoise and orange kingfisher had me dining out for weeks!

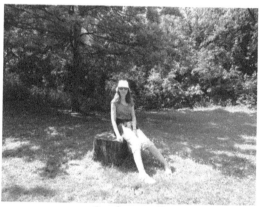

Out for a walk

In Surrey Docks Farm I'd brush past aromatic flower beds full of lavender, rosemary and vegetables, stopping to look at the huge hairy pigs and the clucking, fussing chickens. I'd pick up some of the produce, a marrow, a jar of homemade berry jam and a bunch of flowers. If I ignored the surrounding buildings, my heart lifted, and just for a moment I was back scrumping in Mum and Dad's garden, picking summer fruits with juice running down my chin – eating nearly as many as I put in the basket.

Other poorly people have trod where this farm is now located. Patients with smallpox were transferred from this site to isolation hospitals downriver. On its first night the Blitz largely destroyed South Dock. It became a Fire Service river station and is now an urban farm. Groups of noisy, excited children skipped past often, experiencing a world away from their inner-city school and home life.

My family found it hard to know I was so unwell, living far enough away that they felt helpless. My nature spots gave us something positive to talk about as we caught up on the phone. They came for visits, bringing houseplants and biscuits, a taste of home. We'd exchange hugs but, before the conversation got too close to my illness and the four walls of the flat closed in, I'd suggest we go out. We'd meander towards the river and back again, slowly walking and talking and revelling in the fresh air and much-needed companionship.

Small moments of positivity within the long, grey months kept me going. Friends, colleagues and family sent me bundles of love, emails, cards, flowers and gifts including stripey socks with robins and a postcard of a cat in a woolly hat. Kind visitors drank copious cups of tea with me and distracted me from my illness.

Some days I wanted to hide away, afraid that others would bring my painful emotions to the surface. D's friend would come round for their weekly Xbox night. I'd shut myself away in the bedroom, but Nick would come in anyway and gently, with a few kind words, bring me into the real world. I found it easy to become detached from reality whilst my life had been put on hold.

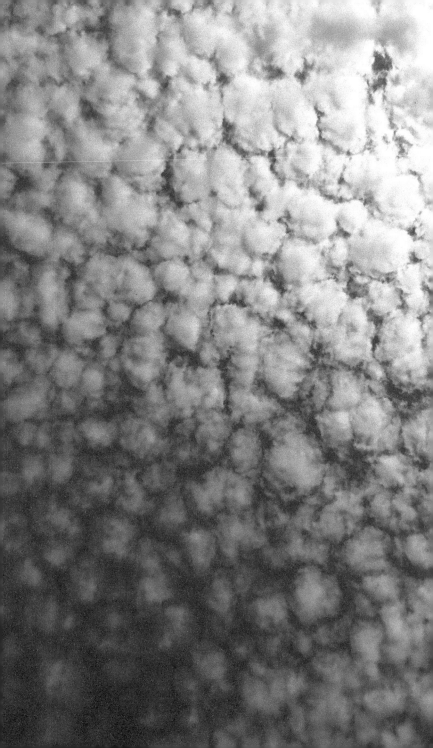

Chapter 7

A longside my nature walks, I sought out other alternative therapies. Cranial osteopathy is a refined and subtle treatment that encourages the release of stresses and tensions throughout the body, including the head. The sessions were somewhat unnerving but effective. As the osteopath placed his hands on my feet, heat crept through my hips, back and all around – as if I had placed a hot water bottle there. His gentle, simple touch probed my nervous system, cradled it and helped it to heal.

I asked him to explain what he thought was wrong. He used the analogy that if my problem had been a skin complaint, it would be like an exceedingly painful red-raw scab that couldn't be touched. Something had made my nervous system hypersensitive to touch and particular sounds.

He gave some holistic advice, and I became obsessed with marginal health gains. I gave up eating wheat because, apparently, that can help with neurological conditions. I gave up caffeine and alcohol. I walked on grass with bare feet to ground myself. I stopped using toiletries and household cleaners with perfumes or parabens. I'm not sure that any of these measures particularly helped, but they gave me a sense of control over the situation. I had been so wretched that I'd try virtually anything.

I saw an acupuncturist to further desensitise my nervous system and speed my recovery. I ventured in with trepidation at the first appointment only to be cocooned in comforting and uplifting aromatherapy scents. After going through a health questionnaire, I nervously let the needles be put in. After she put a large one somewhere in my chest, I burst into tears and sobbed my eyes out. All at once I'd been freed from the fear and tension that I had been holding on to so tightly, and this great unlocking of emotion overwhelmed me.

I travelled home in a daze, all the way from Victoria, heading east to South Quays on the Tube. I dozed and slumbered for twenty-four hours, followed by a sense of relief. The appointments gradually got more manageable and helped dampen my nervous system. Years later, needles helped me to conceive. Being in a heavenly-scented treatment room introduced me to aromatherapy. It's such a lovely way to influence your mood or perk yourself up.

Like a bird you can't identify from its distant song, my illness didn't yet have a name and couldn't be seen. My emotions raged like a storm hitting the coast, casting debris and changing the landscape forever. In the end, the clinical tests came to an end and the day of my next appointment arrived.

Again, we entered the neurology clinic with trepidation. What were they going to say?

I sat down and took a deep breath, holding D's hand. With pleasantries out of the way, the consultant informed me, 'It's good news. The tests haven't found anything wrong with you.'

Silent tears immediately rained down. If there was nothing wrong with me, how could I be fixed? He seemed taken aback at my frustrated sobbing and assured me that it was a good thing that I didn't have any of the conditions he diagnosed in others. As an afterthought, he sent me to a neuropsychiatrist. The weeks in between the two appointments stretched out and thoughts went through the maze of my mind, meeting dead end after dead end, and never quite reaching the centre. I continued to focus on rebuilding my life, and getting out of the maze, one step at a time.

The neuropsychiatrist told me that I had a functional movement disorder (also known as functional neurological disorder or FND), which was likely to be psychological. The symptoms, like my twitching, came from the body not functioning because of faulty brain signals, rather than structural changes. I had a diagnosis, but whilst I now had a name for it the path back to good health wouldn't be easy.

Had I been diagnosed earlier – before I'd found my own way through – the hospital would apparently have provided occupational therapy, psychiatry and physiotherapy. By the time they told me what was wrong, I was already sorting myself out by other means. Happy for me to continue on my own path, they discharged me.

The journey to diagnosis had been highly stressful. If I'd been told from the offset what was wrong, then I doubt it would have got so bad. For me, uncertainty bred anxiety and depression, and this in turn made the FND worse. The NHS is good at ticking things off lists and, of course, this needs to be done. Many doctors admit that they are good at treating illness but often can't help people who are unwell with something that is not adequately understood.

Still physically in crisis, the doctors left me to wait for this glitch or imbalance to evaporate. I wrote in my blog, Even though I know it will go away, not knowing when it will end is quite difficult to deal with. Sometimes I feel like my life is in limbo and that the weeks are stretching in front of me, endlessly ...

I came across only one other person suffering from something similar. In speaking to her my sense of isolation eased and I no longer felt quite so alone.

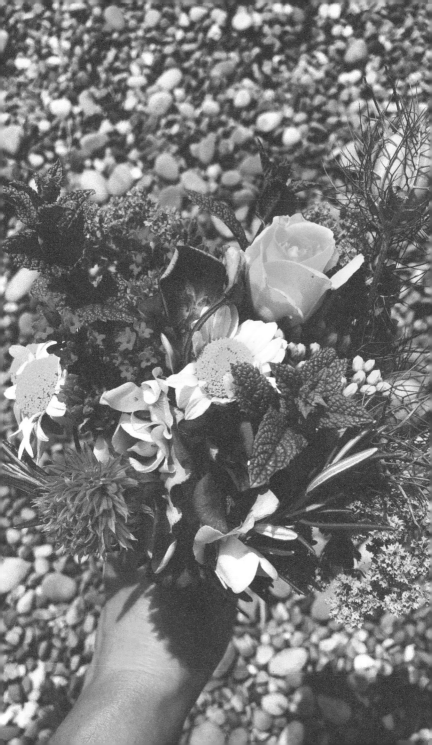

Chapter 8

I went back to the counsellor who had helped lift my depression years previously. We discussed anything and everything to try and get me well again. I pushed against her efforts and like a wounded animal snapped, 'Why me? Other people have worked hard. Why aren't they ill?' She told me to accept my illness and make friends with it. For the first time in my life, I hated my body. Not what it looked like – there were no complaints in that regard. I didn't like how it had behaved and I had lost control.

Lots of people are wary of going to see a counsellor, a therapist, a shrink. They have visions of the tough New York shrinks seen in movies. They think it's not for them. They don't need help. They don't want to drag up their past.

Counselling has definitely improved my life. I went for several years after the series of bereavements in 2001 and have returned more than once since.

It's brave to admit you need help and scary to take that first step. But when you do, you have someone on your side. Someone who knows only what you tell them. They are professionally trained to listen and guide you through their process, which will vary depending on their training and specialisms. I sought help from a Jungian psychoanalyst, psychotherapist and counsellor – simply because on her website it said bereavement counsellor.

During those first sessions in 2001, she would just sit and let me speak. Nothing came out, and it felt awkward. She would ask what had popped into my head. Sometimes I had no words, only tears. The early sessions began with a torrent of emotion around the deaths I was dealing with. With those surface emotions processed, we started to explore why the deaths had affected me, and my relationship with loss and endings.

Some weeks I didn't want any more counselling. I pushed against her suggestions of how to accept my feelings and move on. She had to work very hard. In some ways, it got worse before it got better, but I kept moving forward, not letting depression get the better of me. Often, at the end of the session, she would pose a question for my subconscious to consider. I thought I knew the answer, but I'd have vivid dreams or thoughts that would pop up in the days after my appointment, perhaps telling a different story. I had a recurring dream that my teeth fell out one by one. On waking, I anxiously ran my tongue around my gums to check if my teeth remained in place. Apparently, this is quite common and indicates you are going through a period of change.

Surrounded by plants growing up, my family discussed and observed seasonal changes in great detail. In London, this connection stretched and faded. Ever since rediscovering Mother Nature, she has been a constant comfort and motivator, and this bond has only grown stronger.

I'm confident that, alongside the natural world, my trinity of therapy, acupuncture and cranial osteopathy restored my health. I can't be sure exactly which of them helped the most. They provided a support network and weekly visits with caring professionals. This gave me control over the situation and hope that things would get better. With their help, and my determination, the tremors and twitches subsided and I could finally see a positive path forward. Even through the exhaustion I could slowly take on previously impossible tasks. I went for longer and longer without thinking about my health.

This experience forced me to slow down, contemplate and pay attention to my body. I'm not sure I ever really listened previously, battling on even when under par.

My illness marked the beginning of the end of my time in London. Not long after going back to work part-time and working from home, my employer reduced staff numbers, then wound up due to a lack of funding. I happily took redundancy to become a freelancer. The family business (Perrywood) became my first client, and I could work from our London flat to conserve energy. I started to feel very achy right in my bones. Being inside too much had resulted in a vitamin D deficiency. At last, I had a simple diagnosis that was easily fixed with a daily supplement.

In 2011 D proposed and, since he had looked after me so admirably whilst I'd been poorly, I immediately said yes. He actually asked me, 'What are we going to do about getting married?' Being on wind-swept cliff tops near Beachy Head made up for this low-key proposal. We moved to Essex and got married the same year. There my green recovery continued.

In going back to my roots, I reflected on whether my start in life had any bearing on how I ended up so poorly.

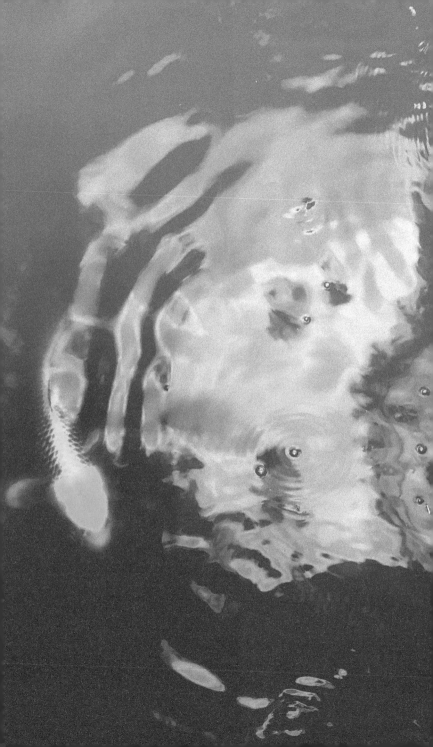

Chapter 9

1977

B orn in Maldon Hospital, Essex, I came out crying. Pulled out with forceps, maybe I just had a headache? During the standard two-week hospital stay, the nurses put me in the linen room because I woke up the other babies with my wailing.

This continued and, at a few months old, in despair, Mum and Dad took me to the local doctor who told them to just let me cry it out. That night they put me to bed in the bedroom next door. I bawled continuously but Dad's chest and heart pounded so much he had to pick me up after just an hour. It took me two to three hours to stop part-sobbing. They put mittens on my hands to stop me from scratching my face as I crossly thrashed around.

Two years later, brother Simon arrived, and four years afterwards Tristan made an early and dramatic arrival. Mum went to the hospital in an ambulance, and Granny looked after us. She nearly burnt the house down after forgetting about a chicken she'd put in the oven. She made a rather short curtain for our back door, and when she put it up Dad kindly said, 'Oh Mik, you've made space for my welly boots.'

Neither Simon nor Tristan had a spell in a linen cupboard. Annoyingly, Simon embodied the perfect baby, although he did rip up my Jack and the Beanstalk book as a toddler. At least Tristan grizzled due to glue ear.

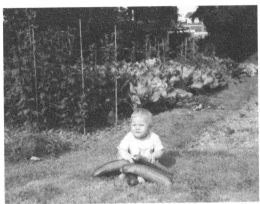

Courgette picking

We went to Sunday school, run by Basil in the local village hall. In one of my school news books (age 6), I wrote that I'd been kept off Sunday school to clean out the garage, and Mum had asked me to put three pairs of knickers in the bin. I can only think something had been lost in translation.

In 1984, a journalist entered our classroom, perching on the small chairs to ask us about our mums.

'Mummy doesn't like it when Tristan cries and wants her,' I said. 'She likes it when we help her tidy up ... she gives us treats sometimes. She says we are her special children.'

My words appeared in the local paper, with my smiling face and straight-across fringe. I did always feel special as a child. As our biggest supporter we always knew whose side Mum was on.

My grandparents, Mary and Les Bourne (Dad's parents), owned a plant nursery and smallholding called Perrywood. We drove the five minute journey regularly to see them as well as Dad, who worked there every day.

I picked up a lot of plant knowledge from Nanny Bourne. I'd often be left with her to give Mum one less child to look after. Walking down the footpaths, she'd point out wonderfully named plants like scarlet pimpernel or broom, encouraging me to look closely and to sniff pineapple weed which magically smelt of the fruit it was named after. We picked flowers for Mum which wilted after twenty-four hours, but the kindness of the gesture lingered.

A field of wheat came up to their bungalow. Our phone would ring, and we'd be told, 'the combine is here, come and watch.' Noses pressed against the window, we'd excitedly see the whirring blades grow nearer, clutching Mum's hand tightly when they looked like they might come through the window. Sometimes we'd be brave enough to venture outside. The smell of combine chaff hanging in the air still takes me back to that place now. I will always get a childlike buzz from seeing a combine or a baler in a field. We'd beg to have a ride on the large two-wheeled barrows, or Nanny and Grandad would ask us to help with simple tasks like lining hanging baskets with moss.

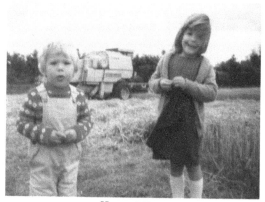

Harvest time

We'd help pick strawberries and would put them in blue cardboard punnets to sell. We'd come home with the sweet taste of juicy sun-baked fruits in our mouths and full tummies. Later we'd enjoy summer pudding, made by Nanny. White bread layered with summer berries in a chipped ceramic pudding dish and left to soak up the juice, served in a thick wedge with double cream – the taste of golden days.

Searching for fruit in Great Uncle Len's raspberry field, I came across a perfect bird's nest. I quietly crept closer hoping to see the fluff of baby birds. Finding it empty, I admired the beauty of the architecture and the simplicity of the building materials – moss, twigs, string and mud – my eyes full of wonder. While my back was turned, Simon tipped my raspberries out of my bowl.

When I was six, we moved to Perrywood and lived in a static caravan for the first winter. We swapped houses with my grandparents, belongings moved by tractor and trailer to the small bungalow where Dad grew up with his two sisters. His bed in the living room had doubled up as a sofa for visitors. His sisters, with a ten-year age gap, had shared a bedroom. The older one would yell, 'Get that brat out of here!' whenever her younger sister wandered in. Mum, very wisely, would not move until the builders had made a start on the extension.

In the mornings we could see our breath in the caravan and, after quickly dressing, walked to use the toilet in the (roofless) bungalow before going to school. I wanted to be lightning quick, to ensure I was not overlooked by the builders arriving on site. My school tights slowed me down, my heart thumped and I couldn't move quickly enough. Baths were also taken under the stars.

Dad could be found decorating until 10 p.m., after a full day's work. After retrieving his shoes from the caravan cupboard, to find them covered in mould, he said to the builders, 'Right, we are moving into the house next week!'

Too young for school, the builders gave my youngest brother chocolate bars out of their lunch boxes, much to my dismay. At school, I couldn't leave the hall until I had drunk the compulsory lukewarm carton of milk and, as one of the last to leave, I missed out on valuable playtime.

Mum had three kids aged six and under and a husband who worked seven days a week. Now I am a parent, I realise just how hard her life must have been. We were signed up for Sunday school because it was the only childcare on offer, rather than for our religious education. I don't blame her for needing a break.

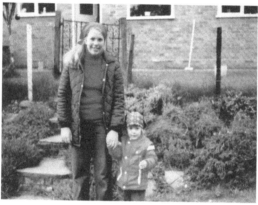

Karin (Mum) and Hannah

When my own daughter was born, she also cried all the time. This is when everyone who remembered my baby years told me with glee, 'Well, that's what you were like. You were awful.'

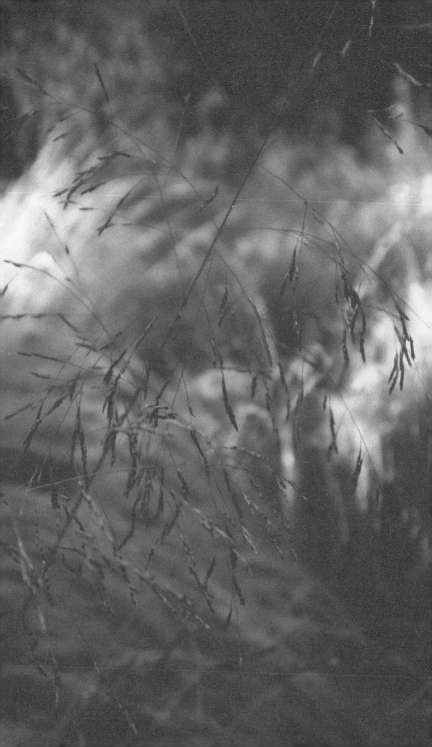

Chapter 10

Not keen to leave Mum's skirts to go to primary school I cried in class during my first week. The teacher sat me under her desk with another tearful child. Not the most auspicious of starts.

I came out of my shell somewhere along the way and performed in several plays. One half of a Dutch pair who performed part of 'A Windmill in Old Amsterdam', singing about a clog-wearing mouse and his antics. We dressed up in full Dutch national clothing, including clogs, depositing Christmas pudding ingredients into a large bowl.

Chosen to appear at a regional school event, I proudly did the actions to 'Auntie Monica', such as swinging my skirt, hat, feathers and my muff. I don't think the last verse is in the songbooks these days. I can't sing particularly well, so I can only assume that I got the gig due to my enthusiasm or a lack of alternatives.

When we returned from a school trip, the headteacher made a beeline for my mum. 'Your daughter is very knowledgeable about plants and nature. We're embarrassed she knows more than us.'

I broke my arm, falling over in the playground. The headteacher was concerned as to how I broke it. 'Did you trip over something?' he queried.

'No, sir, I just fell over.'

Whoops. I am known by my family as 'Hannah Whoops'. Of course, I fell into the water, made the custard far too thick and got bitten on the bottom by my friend's dog, Plimsole. I blame my friend Rachel for that one, though! She wouldn't let me down the slide, so I went back down the ladder and stepped on the dog. In my embarrassment I ran blubbing to my home over the road, unable to tell Mum what the matter was.

On a school trip to Flatford Mill, I crouched by a ditch in my red woolly jumper to recreate a John Constable painting. Excellent execution, but as I stood up in front of all my classmates, my hand felt hot, as if on fire. Ah, nettles on the bank. In looking for soothing dock leaves, I put my hand in dog poo. Whoops.

On a school coach returning from the Norfolk coast, I sat on a newly purchased souvenir windmill magnet and promptly broke it. Whoops.

I have never been a person of precision. I am an optimist, so in my mind, everything will be fine. I carry on regardless. I used to approach my health in much the same way.

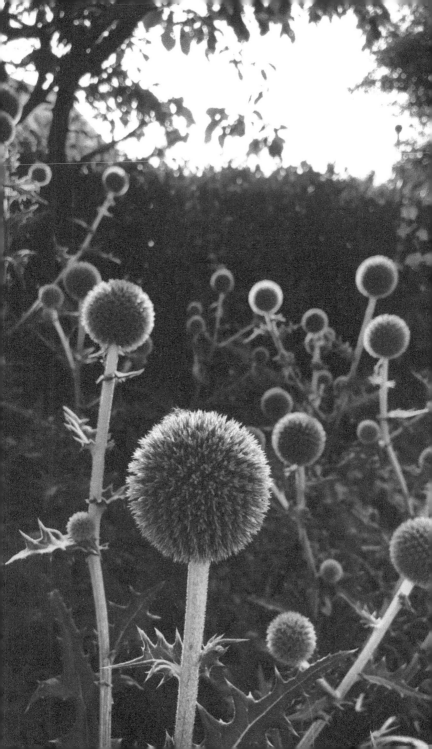

Chapter 11

'Where's Dad?' is probably a familiar phrase in many households. In ours, invariably, the answer was 'outside.' With acres of garden centre, greenhouses and fields to roam, he could be anywhere.

A bell ringer sat on the end of the house, underneath a bedroom window, its button in the shop. We pressed it once for help on the tills, and, to get Dad's attention, we pressed it three times. On a typical evening, I pushed and held three times and waited. He didn't appear, so Simon cycled to tell him to come in for dinner. He didn't return, so Tristan followed on his bike. Eventually, all three trooped back inside, filthy with diesel and detritus from a job that needed doing urgently. Often we started eating without him.

> *A daddy is a squeezy thing*
> *He likes to hug and tickle*
> *In his bath, he sometimes sings*
> *But often gets in a pickle.*
> *But I would really like to say*
> *Have a wonderful Father's Day*
> **Hannah, age 6**

After school, I'd charge upstairs to get changed and then race outside to find something to do. In the spring, we'd 'prick out', the process of transferring tiny seedlings from one big tray into individual pots. I'd found my first money-making job. On planks or boards atop rickety trestles sat a flowerpot full of stones and an empty pot. As I pricked out a seedling, I moved a stone into the empty pot, and at the end of my 'shift' received 1p per plant transfer. I didn't count mowing the lawn for my grandpa as a money-making job. He paid us in Glacier Mints for tending his two-metre-long lawn.

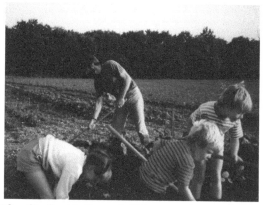

Alan (Dad) with Hannah, Tristan and Simon (L to R)

Dad and I often went out in the van together, and I proudly climbed up to sit next to him. He usually wore nurseryman-green clothes and grubby jeans and, in the autumn and winter, his infamous wax coat and hat. He had brown boots with yellow laces and wore clothes and shoes into the ground until Mum insisted he threw them away or cut them up for rags. He had a full black beard, which made me very suspicious after reading The Twits.

Dad would burn nicotine shreds in the greenhouses to kill pests. He'd light them with a match whilst holding his breath and then retreat. We'd lurk by the door of the glasshouse or, if he'd left us in the house, he'd ask us to come and check that he was okay if he didn't return.

After school, at weekends and in the holidays, Dad and I went further afield. Off we drove to collect conifers from Jack, shrubs from Richard, bedding plants from Roland, polystyrene trays from Derek and chrysanthemums from George. Dad had to seek out and collect plants and cut flowers to sell and I often heard Dad dispensing advice to these other businesses. He didn't hold back if he thought they might be doing something wrong.

Picking up George's big blousy blooms, we'd fill the van with buckets. In them erupted fireworks of yellow, red, pink, orange and copper flowers with a distinctive earthy smell.

I loved entering the local cut flower wholesalers. Joyful flowers came in huge bundles, surrounded by a layer of brown paper or lying flat in cardboard boxes. We'd pick out dark blue irises with streaks of golden yellow, frothy white gypsophila or carnations in a whole host of clashing colours. The warehouse smelt fresh and delicious, especially if pale yellow freesias were in the mix.

We'd collect unwanted cardboard and wooden boxes from the local greengrocers to give to our customers. They smelled of overripe fruit, but sometimes we unearthed a whole, untouched cauliflower or cabbage to take home.

I'd also help out my Aunt Marion. We'd sit on wobbly stools with hard plastic tops across the potting bench from each other, pricking out bedding plants, or brandish our bums in the air as we bent down to pull weeds up during the summer holidays.

My brothers sometimes did these jobs but more often carried out different tasks, utilised for their strength rather than skill. They'd bag up gravel and Growmore, unroll turf so it could be watered, tape up bundles of canes and lift huge 300 litre bales of peat.

Workers Gill and Joyce became like surrogate aunties, often on hand to share their work with me. They even took me swimming but told me off for going underwater as it made them worry.

These three ladies - Aunt Marion, Gill and Joyce - and others along the way, taught me a lot about being part of a team and connecting with people. I learned how to have conversations whilst keeping busy and how to work in companionable silence. We chatted about local events, dinner plans or pets, and, as I grew up, the conversation did too.

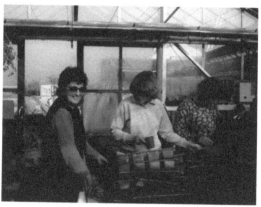

Gill, Joyce and Marion (L to R)

When asked to go through the seed potatoes and take out any rotten ones, I'd begrudgingly oblige. Have you ever smelt a rotten potato? It's like a small animal has died in a confined space. I feel ill just thinking about it.

I liked using the price guns, and I always loved the responsibility of operating the tills, although you had to watch out for the drawers flinging open on the older ones. I also enjoyed using the machine which taped a plant to a bamboo cane – pulling the tape around before stapling it in place.

The teenagers I worked with greeted me with an 'alright' or a nod in school corridors or in the village. It raised my currency, in my eyes at least, especially if they were good looking.

Now I'm a parent myself, I realise that I had to follow Dad around to spend time with him. He told me recently that, when dropping me at Brownies one evening, he said to the other parents, 'I can't wait for Hannah and her brothers to grow up and leave home.' Apparently, we cramped his style. Like his father, he has always wanted to do things his way. It's one of the things I love about him. As a child, I precociously told a team member, 'My daddy wouldn't like you to do it that way.'

I became known as Dad's shadow. Following him around certainly helped my work ethic, which allowed me to be successful in my career, even if it didn't turn out so great for my health - which nobody could have foreseen.

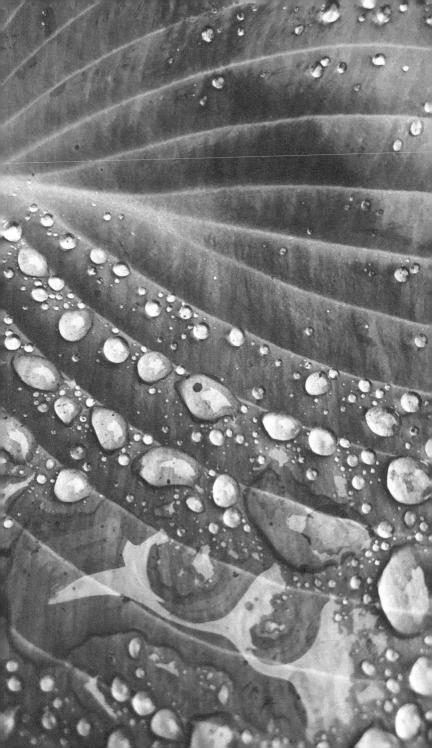

Chapter 12

I never talked to my school friends about plants or mentioned much about where I lived. I didn't want to be the lone bright red poppy in a field of cornflowers. We didn't have loads of play dates as Mum and Dad were so busy working.

Simon and Tristan – generally referred to as Si-Tristan, Tris-Simon or 'the boys' – and I were pretty much allowed the run of the land. We spent days in the 'Ditch Den' – a dry ditch which we commandeered during the summer months. Or 'The Coke Can' – an old water tank on its side which we filled with 'furniture': discarded wooden boxes and other rubbish. The den could be found 'up the top', referring to the top of the site, furthest away from the house. Free and independent, we had our own secateurs and spent hours hacking back the hedgerow. Mum and Dad were very encouraging of our efforts, as it kept us busy and out of trouble.

On hot summer days, we cooled off in the 'swimming pool' - a big metal water tank. The tank was super deep and we couldn't touch the bottom, so I liked to be within reach of the side, and it had a black plastic liner, so we couldn't see anything past our feet. My friend Rachel jumped at the chance to join us and thought it was wonderful we had a swimming pool! We climbed up the stepladder and, as I reluctantly slid into the freezing water, I tried to look brave. When we got out and changed, our swimming costumes would be full of water insects, some of them still wriggling.

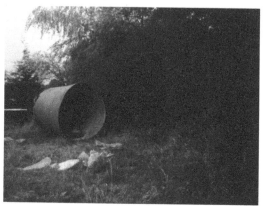

The Coke Can

Simon, Tristan and I would screech with joy as we slid down builders' sand heaps, which doubled up as sandpits, dug vigorously with spades or Tonka diggers. Climbing up towers of peat bales, we'd jump or slide down to investigate the building site of the day. Dad bought us bows and arrows and we cobbled together our own once they broke. We'd ride our bikes around endlessly every day. Up and down the gravel car park or along narrow nursery paths, trying to avoid plants, pots and people as they appeared in front of us.

The three of us caught, counted and released tadpoles. We kept a few in fish tanks and watched them grow legs before putting them in the pond. We collected insects and kept them in jars but we'd ride over the bright green poplar hawk-moth caterpillars on our bikes, because they stripped the leaves off the trees.

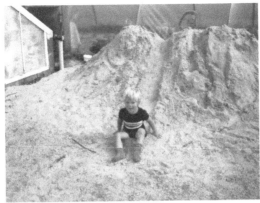

Tristan

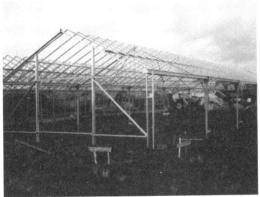

Another building site

Once, we kept some baby rabbits in a box in the garage until they all jumped out and escaped. Our mouser, Pickle, gave birth to her kittens on our doorstep, purring whilst I stroked her tummy during contractions. A brilliant hunter, she had the habit of bringing animals back from her pursuits. She paraded her kills through the garden centre and some customers screeched and complained, especially if she brought back half-dead specimens.

We've had three dogs. Ginger-haired Meg with fluffy ears and paws, the gentlest dog I have ever met, readily available with a cuddle or a nuzzle when I felt sad or out of sorts. She died after local dog food was possibly contaminated. Having lost my friend with no warning, I was inconsolable and took the day off school.

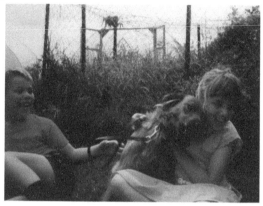

Simon and Hannah with Meg

Then we had Tilly, the crazy Border collie. She chased anything that moved, and she never stopped running. She would follow the tractor mowing the field until the driver stopped. White legs now stained green, she'd collapse, panting and drooling. The minute the tractor started, she'd bounce up again. She dug up a mole one day and, rescuing it, we stroked its velvety black fur and stared at massive spade-like claws. Both of the boys held and examined it. Then I took it and it bit my finger, so I needed a tetanus injection and nearly fainted. I don't really like needles.

Mat loved Tilly, and she returned his affection. Because she was so light, he'd pick her up and carry her on his shoulder. Once, he chucked her off and, jumping around, removed his t-shirt and cursed. Much to our amusement, red flea bites covered his skin. He stopped picking her up after that.

Big, hairy, soppy Sam joined the family unexpectedly. We found him in a hedge outside our house after our neighbour investigated an odd noise. He thought he could hear a baby crying but instead came across a tiny ball of black fluff, whimpering and shaking every time a car went past. We successfully begged Mum and Dad to keep him and named him after Pete Sampras, who had just won Wimbledon. The petite ball of fluff grew into a sizeable flat-coated retriever, possibly with a bit of spaniel thrown into the mix. He couldn't get physically close enough to us, and loved sitting on my feet. He got big enough to jump up and put his paws on Mum or Dad's shoulders, but the sound of vehicles still scared him.

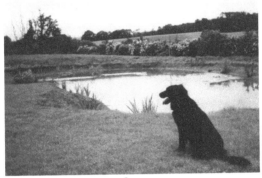

Sam

Our kitchen window overlooked a bird table from which hung a motley selection of broken feeders not good enough to sell. I perched there often to sit and watch the birds, and to keep half an eye on the cars coming in and out of the garden centre entrance.

Birds come and go and, all looking alike, who knows whether they are the same ones returning each day, week, month or year. One distinctive visitor turned up regularly: a blackbird with half his upper beak missing, 'Look, Beaky is back'.

Observing my old friend alongside blue tits, great tits and, with luck on my side, a bullfinch with its pinky-red chest, I sat and thought. Not always about anything in particular, but it was a space where I could organise my feelings about the week just gone, or the one coming up. As I grew older, my attentions increasingly turned to the future. What might it be like to not live here? What would I study, and where?

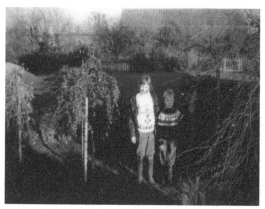

Hannah and Tristan feeding the birds

I always thought I would have a job in horticulture. In fact, cactus surgeon was my earliest aspiration. At the age of six I would sit at this same window, the plants and trees outside, like me, a bit smaller than they are now. Plants lived on the windowsill in front of me, including prickly or hairy cacti. I would gouge out pieces of rotten cactus or sever limbs. I commandeered cocktail sticks from the kitchen drawer in the futile hope of grafting one piece of cactus to another or to prop up a sagging extremity. I dreamt that in the future I would do great things with these weird plants. Sadly, my efforts with the knife were rarely rewarded. My family humoured me and, being only six, I moved on from this pastime with little fanfare. Instead, I concentrated on other things, like quietly standing outside the toilet and making my brother jump when he opened the door to me saying 'boo' very loudly. I also grew proficient in dishing out forearm burns, nips and pinches.

Our parents didn't have the time or energy to pre-assess all of our childhood diversions, and we had a few near misses.

I learned to drive in a Honda Acty truck which I'd rag really fast around the field. Dad bought it to use as a motorised wheelbarrow, but when the garden centre gate closed we children thought of it as ours. Pale yellow, with an open back, it still had the red livery from the dairy who owned it before us. The brakes became decidedly dodgy (non-existent, really). We stood on the back to reach the juiciest blackberries in the prickly hedge, occasionally dropping one down to Sam, who loved them as much as us.

Once, as I drove along for fun, a greenhouse suddenly became rather close in front of me. I had no time to turn. I pumped the brake in desperation and thought about how angry Mum and Dad would be. About to close my eyes and resign myself to an accident, the bonnetless truck and the windscreen and my face came to a stop ... just two inches from the panes of glass. A lucky escape. Simon told me he nearly killed Tristan in the same truck but not to tell Mum and Dad.

Another afternoon Simon cycled down the hill in the field next door, whizzing along the tractor tracks, with feet off the pedals and hidden from view by the tall green shards of wheat. Suddenly he heard a tractor coming into the field – but would the farmer see him before he made it to safety? He pedalled back as fast as he could and he didn't venture back into the field for a while.

Mum and Dad bought the field next door when we started to run out of space for all the greenhouses. The farmer took one last crop of wheat, leaving them the bales. We took the tractor up and down the field to collect them and stacked them up high on the trailer. The whole family was helping or investigating when the bales suddenly fell off, falling and bouncing in two different directions. They hadn't been stacked very well but, thankfully, no one got hit - another lucky escape. When we helped harvest potatoes, we stood on the trailer being pulled along behind the tractor. The trailer didn't have a back and, once, Simon stepped backwards and fell off; luckily, only his pride was hurt.

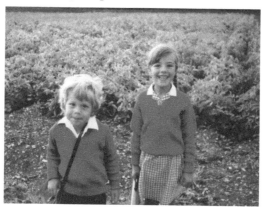

Simon, on his first day at school, with Hannah

When Mat rotavated the soil next to the pond, we heard a splash, some swearing, then silence. His mum and colleague, Gill, ran like the wind down to the pond, terrified that he had fallen under the turning blades. We followed and arrived to see Mat standing up to his waist in the pond, rather sheepishly holding the rotavator in front of him. Gill gave him a right ticking off for scaring the pants off her.

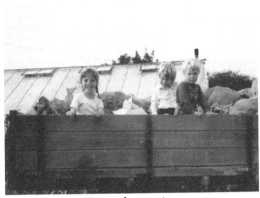

Potato harvesting

I didn't consider working anywhere else when I wanted a regular weekend job and I already had plenty of experience. I was knowledgeable and confident, perhaps at odds with the awkwardness of being a teenager and finding my way at school and with friendships. Put me in the plant area, and I became a brighter version of myself, who could talk clearly and give advice to customers. They looked very unsure that this gangly-looking 14-year-old could be very helpful. I'd start talking and mention a few Latin names, and they'd relax; I'd got the sale in the bag. If I wasn't in the plant area, I could be found on the tills.

At the end of each day, we'd sit around the pine kitchen table and discuss the day's events. We were not shielded from much. Dad shared how he had told someone off for throwing a frog, another for chucking a bat in the air and hitting it away or, on a more positive note, what the sale of the day had been. We discussed the regular customer banned for his unacceptable behaviour towards the ladies. We talked about someone in the team and their performance – good or bad.

The wooden kitchen table doubled up as the HR office, the war room and where we counted the cash. We took it in turns to count the money in the tills and balance the books. It was, without doubt, one of the dirtiest jobs in the garden centre. My hands always smelt of dirt and metal, and some of the notes could be really grubby. A friend gasped when she saw a £50 note in our house and wanted to hold it. I'd seen plenty.

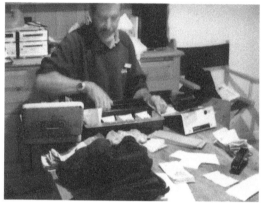

Where we used to count the cash

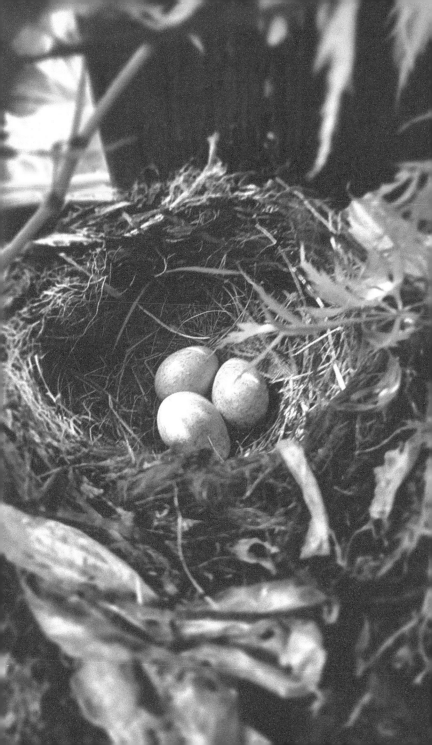

Chapter 13

I was one of only four children to go from our primary school to Thurstable secondary school, in Tiptree. I felt nauseous and on edge for the first few weeks.

Like most children experience, there were many moments where I struggled to fit in. A girl called me Nora Batty for having tights a bit loose around my ankles. Classmates mocked me for my straight-across fringe and growing it out was just as painful. The fringe curled up at the sides, and so now I had wings. I deployed a black fabric Alice band to hide the offending hair, but it took years to fully grow out.

Despite the awkwardness, I had a group of friends who brought much laughter into my life. Sometimes too much. Prone to fits of giggles, the teacher would ask me to stand outside the maths classroom until I could settle down. I'd get myself together and re-enter, only to catch the eye of a so-called mate who pulled a face and set me off anew. Out I went again. Thankfully, I'd moved on from Mr Mendham's class, so I didn't have a blackboard rubber thrown at me.

My report after the first year was glowing. 'Hannah shows a sensible and increasingly mature approach to life and is a pleasant member of the tutor group.' My craft, design and technology teacher gave the most damning feedback – 'She should be aware that overconfidence can inhibit progress.'

Later reports say I was doing well, but wouldn't reach my potential if I couldn't concentrate in class. It's hard to concentrate when you are bored. I would finish the set task and, with nothing to do, I'd join in with the naughty kids or chat and giggle with my mates. We also had some teachers who struggled to keep us all in order.

Our geography field trip took place in the Lake District, and I followed in my father's footsteps, who went on the same journey some thirty-five years earlier. I happily walked the fells and swam in the rivers around Keswick and Borrowdale to measure their width and depth.

Turning up for work experience in a local seed company at fifteen, the office manager told me to go with John to see some specimen plants in his private garden. As I got into his van, I thought that this didn't sound like a great idea. I was ready to hit him and run. Actually, he turned out to be a real gem and a gentleman - an old-school plantsman who loved growing traditional bedding plants. As we opened the greenhouse door, the smell of pungent, musky marigolds hit me like smelling flowers abroad for the first time, under a baking hot sun. I hoed fields with John and his mate, impressing them that I knew one end of a hoe from the other, and collected seeds. We put tomatoes in acid, seeds floating to the top. We stuffed fluffy lettuce seed heads into a machine where you turned a handle to rotate the drum. The heavier seed stayed inside whilst the lighter chaff floated away and made me sneeze. I counted seeds the size of a pinhead inside their lab, using tweezers and a magnifying glass, and it sat with me for weeks that their experiments might be ruined by my lackadaisical counting.

I started to realise there was a world outside Perrywood where other people liked plants and nature as much as my family and me. Even if they were old men, it was a lovely thing to discover.

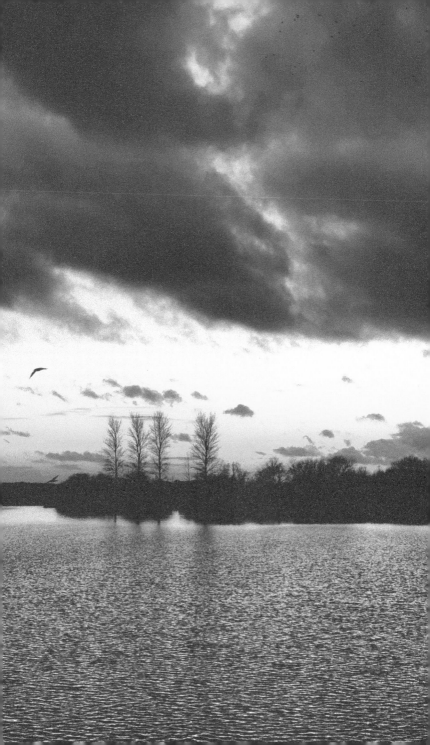

Chapter 14

E very year I looked forward to the Boxing Day walk, normally with my aunt and uncle, Edith and Andrew, and my three cousins. Full of laughter and a cold Christmas buffet, we'd make our way around the same circular walk across the fields. Annually, we reminded ourselves of past pranks and restitched our shared history into the local landscape.

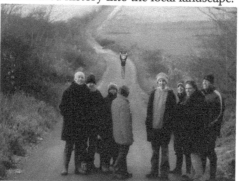

The Bournes and the Richards

'We saw a peacock here once, didn't we?'

'Do you remember, is this where Chris fed Dad a garlic sweet?'

'Who brought that skateboard last year? Isn't this the place Dad rode it into the verge and, as if in slow motion, fell into the grass?'

The mischief popped up at other times of the year, too. One visit, beaming from ear to ear, my cousins proudly presented us with huge homemade Scotch eggs. We wondered why they stared so intently as each of us bit into one. The penny dropped when Dad got mashed potato in his instead of the normal egg.

We travelled to Denmark for many family holidays, where another uncle and other family members lived. We'd stay at a log cabin in the woods and spend hours searching for baby frogs in the long grass, swimming and boating in the warm waters of the lake. Once, I spotted a slow worm slithering across the path in front of me. I quickly skipped and ran to catch up and tell the others, although no one believed me.

We walked through beautiful beech woodlands, which met the beach. One time, leaving footsteps along the golden sands until we realised we had joined a naturist beach. We beat a hasty retreat. On the same walk we stopped for a picnic lunch, whilst waiting for a solar eclipse. I'd been told not to look and didn't want to go blind. As the sun disappeared, I shivered in the suddenly cool air, staring staunchly at the ground. The birds went eerily silent and time stood still. I smiled when the sun reappeared and they restarted their songs.

We visited many relatives who served coffee and Danish pastries. My mum's aunt lived in a house by a lake. We'd take the sloping path down to the water, and it looked big enough to be an ocean, surrounded by swathes of reeds much taller than me. Dad recalled fishing for eels with Mum's uncle, no longer alive. When I think of him, I can smell his pipe, and remember him chatting away in Danish and hoping we would understand. We didn't.

Dad often combined these holidays with work, and we'd visit production nurseries. Acres of dark-green-leaved gardenia stretched out in front of us with their white, sweet-scented double blooms and the same acreage again of orange, red, pink and yellow gerbera daisy-shaped flowers. Even more memorable was the lunch. The nursery owner took us out to a traditional 'Kro' where we all had crispy fried pork and potatoes.

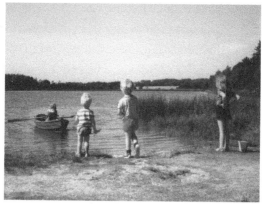

The lake at Slabelle

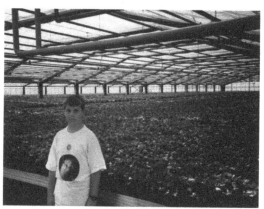

Tristan in front of many Gardenia plants

Djurs Sommerland is etched in our minds. After making decisions about what Dad would carry round for us, we peered at the map of the theme park with its cartoon illustrations of each zone and argued what we should do first. We raced to jump and fall over on bouncy pillows the size of a tennis court, petted or ran away from tame yet boisterous goats, dug in sandpits with sit-on diggers, raced go-carts around a track, panned for gold and pedalled a four-wheeled family 'bike'. But the water raft ride ended in disaster. Tristan hit the back of his head on the way down and finished the ride howling, blood pouring onto his t-shirt. He needed to have his wound stitched and he and Mum headed off in the theme park's small rubbish van stinking of fish, driven by a man in clogs, to see a doctor. Apparently, it was the only available vehicle on site.

In Switzerland to see another uncle, we looked wide-eyed at a plaited manure heap, neat as a schoolgirl's braid. We drank the world's creamiest hot chocolate in a mountain café to the soundtrack of cowbells. We admired a glacier up in the Alps, with its unique blue-and-grey swirls and patterns. Dad found some gentians, a beautiful blue flower which is only found in the mountains. He cradled the deep-sapphire-blue flowers between his fingers, Simon and I next to him as Mum took a picture.

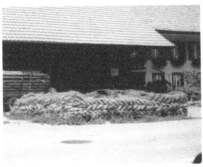

The world's neatest manure heap

In the towns, window boxes full of red and pink geraniums adorned windows everywhere. Uniformly planted, they sang out against the white stone walls and red-tiled roofs. The summer after our holiday, we similarly decked out the front of the house with red geraniums in window boxes and hanging baskets. We chose pink geraniums for the back. They started a new trend locally.

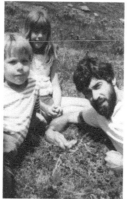

Simon, Hannah and Alan (Dad)

Travelling around England, we visited many of the UK's finest gardens including Bodnant, Dunston, Chartwell, Wisley, Powis Castle and Holkham Hall. We'd often lose Dad and eventually locate him crouched in a flower bed looking for a label (or worse, taking cuttings*) or buying up specimens in the nursery. We'd drive home with hard-to-get-hold-of plants tucked into all available spaces and tickling our legs. Dad would propagate them and sell them the following year. The Welsh tourist village, Portmeirion, captured our imagination with its Italian architecture, hydrangeas, palm trees, fountains and peacocks. So focused on the lush greenery, we lost Tristan for a bit, finding him again after a few panicked minutes.

Living right next to the garden centre, Mum and Dad sought out quieter spots for holidays. One year, they booked a converted cottage on a remote Welsh farm. The farmer took us off-roading across his Snowdonia mountains in our 4WD Mitsubishi Shogun. Dad sat in the driver's seat with his farmer guide next to him. Mum and the boys sat in the back, and I drew the short straw, taking the fold-down seat in the boot. What an adventure. The farmer had such a strong Welsh accent, I couldn't really understand him and just had to hope that Dad understood enough to get us safely across the steep hills. Dad and his navigator tested the Shogun to its absolute limit, taking on sheer inclines and leaving us wondering if we might fall off the edge of the world. Dad looked very at home.

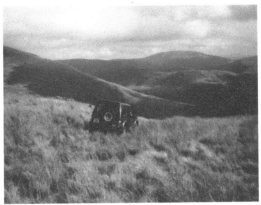

Off roading

Black Rock Sands beat others to become our favourite beach. Dad drove onto the sand and we said 'are you sure we can park here?' Whatever the weather, we spent hours with our nets by the rock pools, catching tiny fish and shrimps. Inland we sought out waterfalls, streams and rivers to paddle, swim and fish in. We strode along the 8.7-mile Roman Steps trail near Llanbedr, gazing at the purple heather and stopping to look over sunny mountain views. The clouds arrived suddenly, and we scrambled to get our waterproofs on. Tristan and I wanted to turn around and descend. Both spooked, the others encouraged us to keep going to the top. I found the energy to bound up the twenty-seven carved steps, for which the trail is named, probably cut by workers at the now-disused quarry. Dry from the rain, I quickly became sweaty in my cheap, red jacket. The clouds disappeared as quickly as they came. We bundled Macintoshes away again and, in the sunshine, we stopped for fish paste rolls, wine gums and a swig of water.

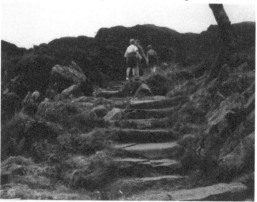

Up the Roman Steps

As a teenager, I completed my Bronze, Silver and Gold Duke of Edinburgh awards. I enjoyed the expeditions the most. My friends and fellow walkers would ask me to identify plants on our way past trees, hedges and wildflowers. We had fun and it helped us pass the time. They later admitted that they'd hoped they'd find something I didn't know. The Gold practice expedition in the Brecon Beacons didn't go to plan. Being in Wales, it rained and blustered rather more than was normal in Essex. On the first day, we tied ourselves together with rope as we traversed the hills because we didn't want our smallest team member to get blown away, a real prospect. The storm drenched us through, so we all sat in the campsite laundry room in our undies to dry our sodden clothes. The next day we were slow to get going. We struggled to pack away our tents in another downpour, fingers becoming numb with cold, rain sluicing down coats and finding a way to trickle inside, down arms and necks. Soaked through again the packs felt heavier than ever.

Being behind schedule, we missed the turning down to the bottom of the valley and our campsite and instead found ourselves atop the mountain at dusk. Not realising, we kept walking on narrow paths with a sheer drop to one side. One of my teammates feared heights and kept stopping to cling to the ground, softly moaning in terror. I'm not a massive fan of heights myself and couldn't do much to help. As the sun disappeared behind the peaks, we admitted defeat and decided to do as we were trained: set up camp and stay there until first light.

An unplanned camping trip at the top of a deserted mountain is not to be recommended. We could see and hear a helicopter searching for us and flashed SOS signals with our torches but, frustratingly, it never quite came close enough.

Fighting back fear and tears, Rachel and I refused to camp alone, so we squeezed into a tent, head to tail, with three 16-year-old boys. What started as a good idea ended with a lot of farting, smelly feet and giggling, and not enough room. Sleep did not come easily and we didn't wake until the sun had fully risen. When we eventually roused, we blearily opened the tent to see a tiny campsite in the valley below, nowhere we had expected it to be. We trekked down expecting our teacher to be delighted to see us alive. Instead, she bellowed at us, 'Where the hell have you been?'

Had we risen at first light, we would have made it down a lot earlier. Our worried teacher had been preparing to call our parents, deciding not to get in touch with them the previous evening. We grumbled all day about her apparent lack of concern.

These experiences cemented my love of the natural world. Away from the classroom, I could be myself in jeans and a fleece jumper and enjoy nature's bounty. I discovered a wider, inspiring world far away from my everyday teenage worries and struggles.

he was very naughty. I promise he has not done this for many years.

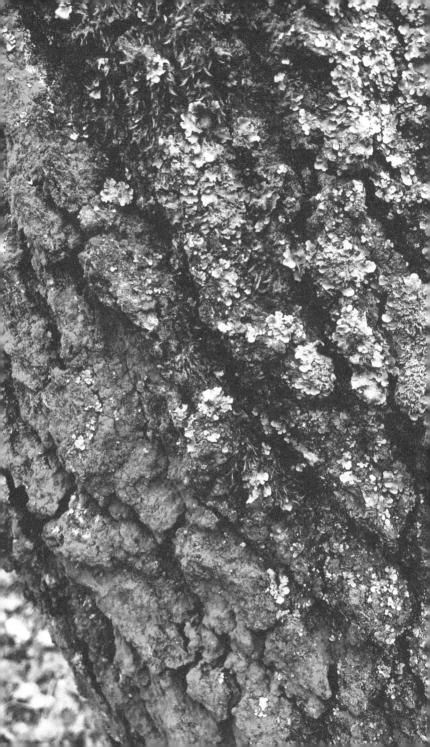

Chapter 15

I didn't really consider doing anything else but study for a horticulture degree. There were only six colleges and universities to choose from. I'd have no independence if I went to Writtle in my home county of Essex, and I discounted two more.

Mum, Dad and I visited Hadlow College and two universities, Nottingham and then Reading. Dad in particular loved having a nose around their greenhouses and gardens, generally found at least 100 metres behind the guided tour. He peered through doors that said 'Private' or bent down to glance under a plant bench, having a closer look at something or other.

The campus at the University of Reading, where I ended up, began life as an agricultural college, which explained the many remarkable trees. The thought of moving there and not knowing anyone gave me a hollow feeling in the pit of my stomach. I packed my bags and took a last look around the garden centre, saying goodbye to the team and saving up a library of images in my mind.

Homesickness hit, but I was having too much fun to pine too much. Once a week I queued up to use the public cash phone, hoping that someone at home would answer. Mum and Dad kept me informed of the latest family and garden centre news, shortening the distance between us. My brothers were still at school, and our chats were brief, having little in common.

I became great friends with my corridor 'housemates' in Wells Hall. On one hand, I revelled in meeting people from different backgrounds and, on the other, was reassured to meet others like me. In the Wells Hall bar, I drank five pints of lager and lime on a 'quiet night', and played darts and pool extremely badly. I'd then go up to our tiny kitchen to cook pasta, which soaked up all the alcohol and made up for yet another disappointing dinner from Martin the Chef. We didn't really blame Martin when we learned how little budget he'd been given for each meal.

At the weekends, I drank even more. We'd have a bottle of wine each before heading out to a bar or club. In the student bar, snakebite and blacks were lined up, knocked back with abandon. Later on, tequila or other foul-tasting shots did the rounds. In the clubs, we'd drink alcopops, sugary-sweet, like drinking squash. We'd all get drunk every weekend. Apart from one lad who went home at the weekends because he didn't trust his parents to look after his cat. Or so he told us. Maybe he just didn't want to hang out with a load of pissheads. On Sunday mornings, we could be found in McDonald's, wearing sunglasses whatever the weather, studiously ignoring the children screaming in the soft play area and hoping the McMuffin breakfasts would sort us out. If I couldn't face going out, I'd go to the local shop, making do with a can of Lilt and a large packet of salt and vinegar McCoy's crisps.

Jim, our halls warden, was a botany lecturer, a dedicated pipe smoker and a dead ringer for actor Leslie Nielsen. At a summer BBQ, he asked if anyone could name the tree in front of us. My friends all looked at me and I told him it appeared to be some kind of ash. He smiled and said he always asked his botany students this question. Most people incorrectly guessed it was an oak. I won a bottle of beer for my efforts.

In my first term, our tutor took us into a potting shed and showed us how to sow sweet peas. Inwardly, I thought, 'Hey, I did this at five years old.' The following week we removed leaves from a patch of grass, working out the comparable efficiency of the leaf blower versus the rake. Again, I thought, 'This is so boring!'* I enjoyed new subjects such as entomology, botany and even statistics, definitely not a breeze. I'd have liked to come across more students like me, potty about plants. I had no green-fingered tribe to hang out with but did get to visit Norfolk vegetable farms. I felt only mildly jealous on hearing a school friend had travelled to Spain for her university field trip.

More excitingly, we went by bus to Kiftsgate Court Garden in the Cotswolds. There, a summer house perched on a hill below the main house. I ran inside for shelter in a sudden downpour and sat on a swing seat, looking out over the garden. My stomach flipped when a guy I fancied did the same and sat next to me. It could have been the romantic moment I'd been hoping for. Instead, we sat and listened to the rain, chatting about this and that, before moving on after the clouds passed. The atmosphere had become humid, steam rising as the sun hit the wet plants and paths. The star of the garden was the musky-scented Kiftsgate rose; a truly remarkable sight. Thousands of white blooms covered several trees in front of us. I forgot about my potential suitor and stood and stared – a moment to savour.

Come the end of term, I headed home to revise for my exams. I tried to study in Mum and Dad's conservatory but couldn't get over my drowsiness and kept falling asleep. I blamed it on sitting in the sun and did my best to push through. I returned to Reading where, entering one of the exam rooms, I felt headachy, shaky and sleepy. A member of staff kindly drove me to the university medical centre, where I was told I had glandular fever. I resided there for the rest of my exams, sleeping in a small private room. Several of us sat in the same exam room, doing different subjects. We wore our pyjamas; there was no invigilator. At the other side of the room, I saw a girl I recognised, someone I shared lectures with. We made eye contact and smiled, but neither of us considered cheating even though we had been left alone. Despite my weariness, I passed the exams but many didn't, disappearing to their hometowns to reconsider their options.

Year two. We now lived off-campus. To help me save my energy for classes, in my ongoing recovery from glandular fever, Mum and Dad bought me a car to reduce my weekly steps. I missed the meandering walks, the earthy autumnal smell of the leaf mould, and whilst driving I couldn't touch the trunks or look up into the tree canopies.

We visited friends' homes for the weekend or in the holidays. They ranged from normal semi-detached and detached houses in the suburbs to larger farmhouses, a Brussels townhouse and even a Sussex house with a moat and a secret corridor behind a panelled wall. There, I went to the toilet and couldn't understand why the bathroom was even hotter than the summer's day outside. I reached for the soft towel, also warm. I had never seen a heated towel rail before and stored up the experience to tell Mum and Dad when I next called. In a West Country farmhouse, my friend's Mum fed us roast dinner with baked beans, and enough desserts to have one each. My bedroom had been dressed for a day at the races, adorned with a pelmet and frilly bed linen.

Uni friends often introduced me to their parents as 'Hannah Flowers'. I lived with another Hannah and friends needed to distinguish us. The other, of house-with-moat fame, was 'Posh Hannah'.

Invariably, at some point I'd be asked to examine some poorly specimen in their garden. 'What's wrong with that, do you think?'

'That one? Oh, I'm afraid that's dead,' I cheerfully replied.

Before year three I stayed in Reading for a summer because I wanted to gain experience by working somewhere different, to boost my CV. I helped with research into cocoa plants at the university, setting up irrigation systems and pollinating flowers using a paintbrush.

I also got a summer placement at Waterer's Nursery in Bagshot, a wholesale nursery growing shrubs, and I joined in with weeding, pot washing in their dispatch area and pruning. The workers smiled to come across a horticulture student with some practical knowledge and who knew all the Latin names of the plants. I found it reasonably easy to ingratiate myself with my new colleagues and the days were very pleasant.

Coming home to the empty house at the end of each day made me feel very lonely, so I'd phone home each evening to talk to somebody. Princess Diana died that summer, which meant the TV was full of tributes and the radio only played sombre music, which added to my glum mood. I also locked myself out of the house once. Not knowing what to do, I called Mum and Dad, but no one answered. A neighbour brought a ladder around, which fell short of reaching the upstairs open window. He claimed to have experience, which I hoped meant he worked as a fire officer rather than a burglar. I really hoped he wouldn't fall on my account; I held my breath. Heroically, he used his muscly arms to pull himself up to the window and let me in again. I left beer on his doorstep the next day to say thank you, in the misguided hope there might be a romantic ending.

Crammed into our final abode, a terraced house in the middle of town, we craved greenery and open spaces. A few of us had cars, so we'd drive into the countryside for short walks and pub lunches at weekends. We discovered beech woodlands, the river in Henley and Marlow, and Beale Park in Pangbourne, where we saw deer and waterbirds. Trips like these provided a release from the stresses of coursework and an antidote to frantic socialising.

At my graduation, I posed with Mum and Dad in front of beautiful acers, which of course, we commented on. In the ceremony, surrounded by ornate green, gold and cream ceilings and twelve-foot-high organ pipes, we all laughed when one lad's name was read out. His two middle names were Murray and Walker.

Graduation meant the end of an era, and I didn't want friendships or the fun to end. Mum and Dad didn't expect me to come home and work at Perrywood, but a part of me insisted that I should. It was my family's business, and I was the oldest. I loved plants and had a degree in horticulture. Why would I do anything else?

I had a uni friend who, as the oldest son, was due to inherit his father's farm in North Wales. He understood the conflicting feelings of having a fantastic opportunity to follow in your parent's footsteps yet resenting the hold it had over you. It could restrict my life if I let it.

In case you are wondering, I'm pretty sure the rake turned up trumps.

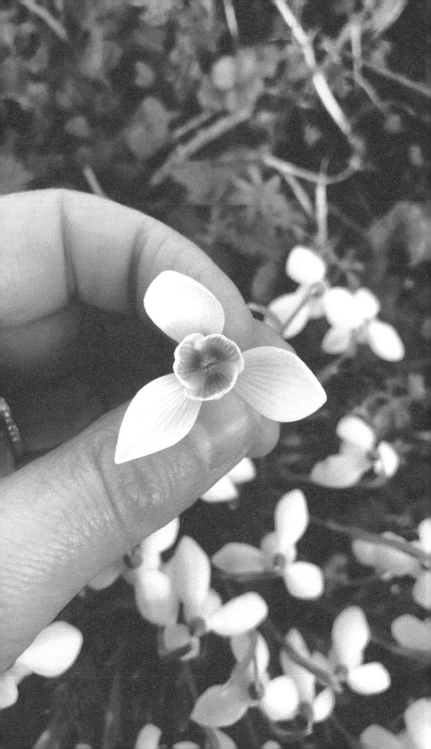

Chapter 16

My holiday jobs at Perrywood having earned me enough money to pay my way through uni, I used my third-year student loan to visit Australia and New Zealand, putting off the decision of what to do next. My good friend Louise and I travelled from Cairns to Sydney, stopping off in all the backpacker haunts.

The prospect of getting up close and personal with coral, exotic plants and strange southern hemisphere animals filled my head as we landed. As we left the aeroplane we got hit in the face by a wall of humid air, and quickly stripped off our extra layers.

On day one, we booked a boat trip out to the Great Barrier Reef. We chugged out to sea and started to feel rather green, taking it in turns to vomit into the boat's tiny toilet. Once moored up, I put on the snorkelling gear, jumped into the water and the nausea disappeared. I put my face down into the water, mesmerised by the underwater scene. A kaleidoscope of colours burst into view, from shoals of tiny, darting fish, weird and wonderful corals and ribbons of seaweed. I ignored how weak my limbs felt and kicked out my flippers, but we had to get back on the boat all too soon.

The minute we stood upright, our seasickness set in once more, and the return journey was utter misery. Leaving the boat with shaky legs and empty tummies, we found the nearest McDonald's and vowed never to go on a boat again. We shared the story with other backpackers that night, and they laughed at us because, apparently, jet lag and boats are not a good mix.

We travelled from hostel to hostel, covering considerable distances in the bus, before breaking our vow to stay on dry land. We hopped on board an ex-sailing yacht for a trip around the beautiful Whitsunday islands, with their turquoise waters, golden silica sands and access to more of the Great Barrier Reef.

We moored up in the middle of the Coral Sea, no land in sight. The captain asked a volunteer to swim around the boat and, as she hit the water, we looked on in amazement. As her feet and arms created currents, the water lit up with phosphorescence, the bioluminescence of tiny organisms in the sea. Returning to the start, she left in her wake a perfect ring of light around the boat. I had never seen anything so incredible until afterwards, when we lay on the boat's deck and looked up to see an inky dark sky crammed full of stars, planets, shooting stars and galaxies. Yet again, my mind was blown, and I felt insignificant, in a good way. Part of something vast and incredible. Whatever the events in my own life, nature and the universe would always be there.

We moored our boat on Hamilton Island for the night, haven for the super-rich. Sitting in the swimming pool, a white-and-yellow cockatiel in the palm tree above caught my eye as it ate a packet of crisps, taking them out one by one with its beak. We revelled in this incongruous sight but the glimpse of a common green turtle whilst snorkelling stopped me in my tracks. It looked at me through wise eyes before slowly and gracefully gliding away.

Springtime bloomed in the southern hemisphere. In Brisbane, we stood under an avenue of jacaranda trees covered in pale purple blossoms; looking up in wonder as petals gently rained down on us like confetti. We took an inland diversion to stay on a dry, dusty cattle ranch, where the sign on the toilet said, 'If it's yellow, let it mellow', to encourage us to save water. The dusty farm grew few trees and plants, and it wasn't somewhere I would rush back to. Likewise, we passed through Surfers Paradise quickly, not enjoying the high-rises, the bling and the frivolousness. Most of the natural world there had been stripped away, leaving only the white sand and blue sea.

Disembarking from the bus in Byron Bay, I instantly felt more at home, surrounded by trees, parks and nature trails. We ended up staying for two weeks, days spent bodyboarding on the beach and exploring the area, and evenings drinking. Recharging didn't mean holding back on the alcohol though. One night I vomited repeatedly from drinking far too much tequila. I just didn't have an off switch and, as much as I regretted it each morning, I knew I would be drinking again that night. It wouldn't be tequila, though, and I have never drunk it since.

I fell in love with the botanic gardens in Sydney. There had been less flora than I had been expecting on the trip to date. A display of cannas with scarlet red flowers and giant green leaves provided the perfect foreground for yet another snap of the iconic opera house. I craned my neck to look up at the fourteen-foot-high agave flowers and grinned at the colossal cactus. Each evening blobs hanging in the trees opened their large leathery wings - fruit bats flying in groups across the sky like the terrifying winged monkeys in The Wizard of Oz.

In Sydney, we stayed in the worst backpackers' hostel of the trip. In a mixed dormitory, I ended up in the top bunk. I went to sleep hot and sweaty, skin sticking to the plasticky sheets, and dreaming of losing limbs because the ceiling fan seemed way too close for comfort. Woken by a noise, I heard a tap running. I blearily looked round, and others did the same, to see one of our room-mates standing in the corner, peeing. We were horrified until we saw he was peeing on his own bag, not any of ours. He didn't respond and was sleepwalking, so we giggled and went back to sleep. No one told him in the morning, and my friend and I left to find another hostel.

Meeting up with another friend from university, we hired a car to explore some of the areas outside of Sydney. I scraped the side of the hire car on a wall as we made our way out of the underground car park. Whoops. In my defence, the exit was very narrow. We stopped in a lay-by to inspect the damage and hunted for a cloth to see if we could rub away the evidence. The only item of clothing we were prepared to sacrifice from our scant belongings? A clean pair of knickers.

I looked forward to leaving the city behind and seeing some Australian countryside. We visited the Home and Away beach and went to the birthplace of Skippy the Bush Kangaroo. Hundreds of kangaroos filled field after field in Waratah Park, many with joeys in their pouches, making them look like weird, multi-limbed creatures. We came across a paddock with one resident, with a sign saying this was Skippy's descendent. It seemed a shame that he'd been ostracised from the rest of the herd because he had a famous relation. I secretly hoped that they rotated the inhabitant occasionally. Three years later I read the park lessee had been charged with animal cruelty and his licence revoked.

Back in Sydney we caught a train to the Blue Mountains, taking everything we owned, which included a large watermelon. We needed all our extra layers in the cold mountain air, but the spectacular views made up for the missing heat. It became my second-favourite spot in Oz, after the Barrier Reef. We stood and gazed over the Three Sisters rock formation and the wide tree-lined canyon. I tried to take in the hectares of blue-green Eucalyptus trees, the sky holding a familiar fragrance reminiscent of cold remedies. I was miniature in comparison. The oil-filled air was hazy - like something out of a book or film. I stood and stared until the others got bored and pulled me away from my reverie.

I reluctantly headed to the airport to say goodbye. I'd be journeying to New Zealand on my own, and suddenly a wave of doubt hit me. I had family there but would be travelling around alone. My friend would soon be reunited with her family and tears streamed down my face after we hugged.

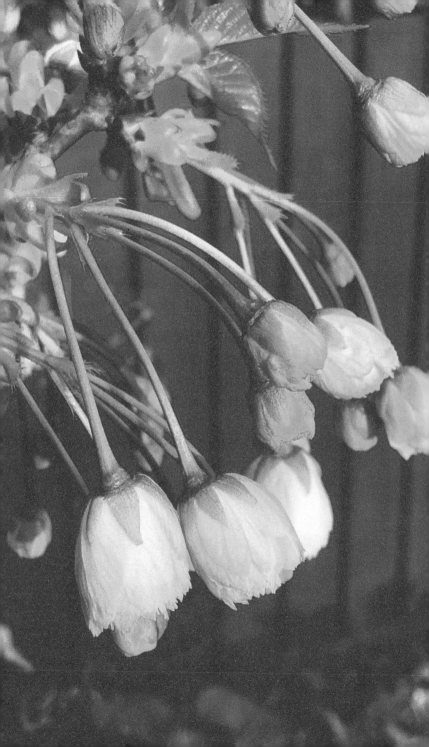

Chapter 17

December 1999

New Zealand, South Island. In Christchurch, roses bloomed, and I bent down to smell a dark red variety, then looked up to see Father Christmas go past in his shorts. This bizarre encounter threw me out of kilter. My bond with the seasons had been turned upside down.

I needed to stop moping, so I booked a guided kayak trip in Abel Tasman Park. The sands shone with golden allure, the water crystal clear, and we whizzed along in kayaks with red-and-purple spinnaker sails stretched out in front of us. I felt on top of the world. We stopped to float awhile, and a seal swam under and around my kayak. As it gracefully pirouetted in the water, I beamed from ear to ear.

My next stop was Kaikoura, for whale watching. I jump up and down at the sight of a new plant, bird or even insect, so I wasn't sure how I would react to seeing one of the world's largest mammals.

In the car park, a West Country voice called out, 'Oi, Bourneo!'. I turned and saw Mark, a Reading alumnus whose booming voice I knew well, being the loudest in lectures. He was leaving Kaikoura that day and I'd just arrived. I didn't think I'd bump into anyone on my travels, but remarkably his was the third familiar face I'd seen on this trip. I was charmed to have had three chance encounters so far from home. We exchanged pleasantries and continued our own journeys, never to see each other again.

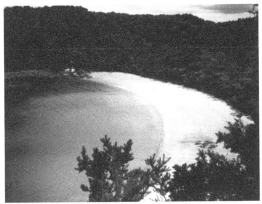

Abel Tasman

Kaikoura sits in a curved bay with a stony beach and mountains coming down to greet the sea. In the boat, we came across a pod of hundreds of dusky dolphins. They entertained us with their jumps, leaps and somersaults, delicately entering the water or purposely slapping it with their sides or backs. They put on a terrific show, and the baby dolphins also held our attention as they swam within a metre or two of the boat.

Further out, we spotted the main prize, a humpback whale. Everyone ran to one side of the boat and I wondered if we might tip over. At first, we saw just the top of its head, and water spraying upwards from the blowhole. Then it lazily dived, its back popping up before the black-and-white tail casually flipped up and out of the water and then disappeared. Below water, it would have been the same size as our boat, yet we only saw a small part of it. I radiated smiles having seen one of nature's largest creatures. Yet, I felt a closer connection to the spellbinding dolphins, the day's unexpected highlight. Everyone returned to shore on a high, bonding over this special shared encounter.

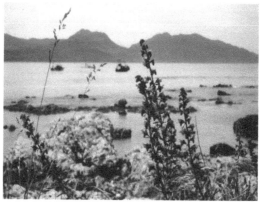

Kaikoura

Onwards to Dunedin, to stay with my Uncle Neil, his partner Anni and their four children. We usually had the nearby breathtaking beaches to ourselves. We slid down sand dunes and paddled in the cold water.

As the adults busied themselves building a house one afternoon, I helped out by cooking tea. Only, I blew their heads off, accidently using cayenne instead of paprika. Whoops. My young cousin, Daniel, wailed, 'I just wanted a proper tea.'

His older sister Ana shares her birthday with the summer solstice. We threw our offering – a figure woven from long flax leaves – into the water before we devoured a raspberry pavlova.

Christmas Day came and went. I was thankful to be able to phone home and find out what had been going on. It felt like I had been away for aeons, but not much had changed back in Essex. Then, on Millennium Eve, Neil and I sat by the fire pit and whiled away the hours until we strolled around the headland with Anni to see the fireworks over Dunedin harbour. A more subdued New Year's than normal. I didn't miss the crush of the crowds, the pressure to find someone for a midnight kiss. Tonight, we really earned the fireworks and after walking back in the early hours, by moonlight, I went to bed tired and content.

They ventured south with me, and in the Catlins we sat in lush grassland reading books, and stood on a clifftop counting the number of waves until the biggest one came round again. I had no idea waves travelled in groups and watched transfixed.

It was a wrench to leave behind a family I had reconnected with, knowing I wouldn't see them again for a long time. Butterflies filled my stomach, and I headed off alone again.

In the loud and vibrant Queenstown, I felt like a forlorn cub missing its mother. I hiked up to the top of a mountain and became a proud lioness, surveying my kingdom. Peter Jackson filmed the Lord of The Rings (LOTR) trilogy here recently, and it was easy to see why – craggy mountains rose forebodingly from the blue lake. Bursts of purple and pink dotted the landscape - wild lupins, the first of many that I'd see throughout this island. I'd always thought them a blousy, showy plant until seeing them in this wild tableau.

Back in town I got my hair cut; a very high mark on the wall showed a recent flood line. My hairdresser told me the LOTR film crew and cast all came to help the town evacuate and move their belongings ahead of the flood. I'd been feeling disconnected, so I enjoyed hearing about some community spirit.

I alighted a coach which wound around roads for what seemed like an eternity, my neck permanently twisted to quickly scan one stunning scene after another through the window. Finally at Milford Sound I could get out and explore, and our boat motored out across the inky blue-black water. Here my head twisted upwards to gaze at the vertical rock faces of the huge mountains enveloping us. Boats looked like toys. A waterfall the height of a skyscraper towered above us. Reluctantly, I got back on the bus, full of the place I was leaving behind.

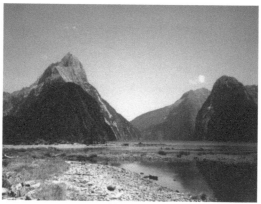

Milford Sound

I joined the West Coast Express, a guided minibus tour from Wanaka to Picton. Strangers quickly became friends and, to my surprise, Helen, the Scottish grey-haired grandmother of the group, was the most fun of all. She joined in with the drinking, laughed the loudest and blasted through my misguided stereotypes of older, retired folk. We explored some of the world's most stunning places. We drank wine in a vineyard that stretched down to the teal-blue waters of Lake Wanaka, hollyhocks punctuating the landscape with their colourful red, pink and yellow flower spikes. We jumped across boulders the size of trucks next to a river. We trekked through prehistoric landscapes, expecting dinosaurs to appear from behind the tree ferns, grey-green mosses hanging down from branches above us. We stood alone on Haast beach, surrounded by sand dunes, pebbles and bleached driftwood, before the sandflies eventually moved us on.

Partway through the trip, we met our tour company's sister bus making the reverse journey, north to south. I hit it off with one of their passengers and had a one-night-only encounter with a handsome stranger in a glow-worm cave. The glow-worms should have been fascinating, but my attention was elsewhere.

Drawing closer to the snow-capped mountains, we hitched a helicopter ride to hike on the Fox Glacier. I sat with the glass windscreen extending beneath my feet, sheer mountain faces and the grey and white glacier displayed in all their glory. I stepped onto the ice in my shorts, with snow crampons attached to my boots. We used poles to test the ground and gingerly followed the guide, marvelling at the weird and wonderful shapes in the ice and looking for, but not seeing, any signs of wildlife. Back to a bar for a drinking game with some old German men – we consumed many steins of beer, and went to bed on a high.

In Punakaiki, we explored an ancient river in kayaks and wondered if anyone had ever been there before. There was no sign of humans from the water, and we could get up close to the green tapestry of trees and plants on the banks. Punakaiki means 'pancakes', and the rock layers alternate between limestone, made of tiny shell fragments, and siltstone. Thousands of years of sea, rain and wind have eroded the softer siltstone, leaving the limestone layers looking like a stack of pancakes.

Under the silent, watchful gaze of the age-old, worn rocks we gathered on the beach. With sandy toes, sunburnt noses and salt-tangled hair, we watched until the burnt-orange sun disappeared over the Tasman Sea, trailing in its wake a sea and sky flecked with pinks and lilacs as from a summer meadow. Back sitting on white plastic hostel chairs we invented Punakaiki Punch, a potent drink made of peach schnapps, rum and fruit juice. Under its influence we went for a night-time walk, instead stopping to lay on the ground and look at the incredible southern hemisphere stars. We lost our way in the dark and stumbled around laughing until the clever one with the head torch guided us home.

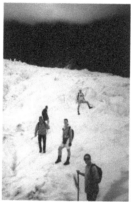

Fox Glacier

Onward towards our last stop, Picton. We lay down again, all on top of each other, for a cheesy picture. Later that night, in between pubs, we posed on the train tracks like we needed rescuing. The tracks were not live, and whilst the rail safety video from my school days entered my mind, we knew the next train would not be for hours. I left my new friends behind to continue exploring, wondering if I would ever see them again.

I joined a group of tourists picked up by boat and dropped off next to the Queen Charlotte Track in the Marlborough Sounds. In finding my own pace, I lost the others to walk alone, in this magical dreamlike place. The by-now-ubiquitous tree ferns towered above me, making shadows on the path, their light green fronds shading me from the heat of the midday sun.

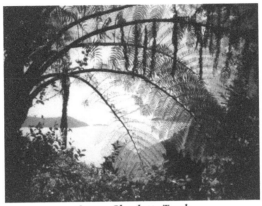

Queen Charlotte Track

The sea view on my left-hand side came and went. The sweet-smelling white flowers and tiny, dark leaves of Manuka bushes held my attention as my feet carried me forward. Later I learnt the Manuka plant is the source of tea tree oil, so named because Captain Cook and his crew boiled the leaves for tea and, seemingly, not much had changed round here since they explored. The chiming of bells preceded the arrival of olive-green-feathered bellbirds, whilst black-and-blue-green tame tui, having no predators, regularly flew down to land in front of me and show off their white throat tufts. There were no vehicles, no people; just me, the birds and their unfamiliar yet uplifting song. Immersed in this montage I forgot the loss of my bus mates. I wanted to stay there forever, and was disappointed when the boat picked me up after the day's walking.

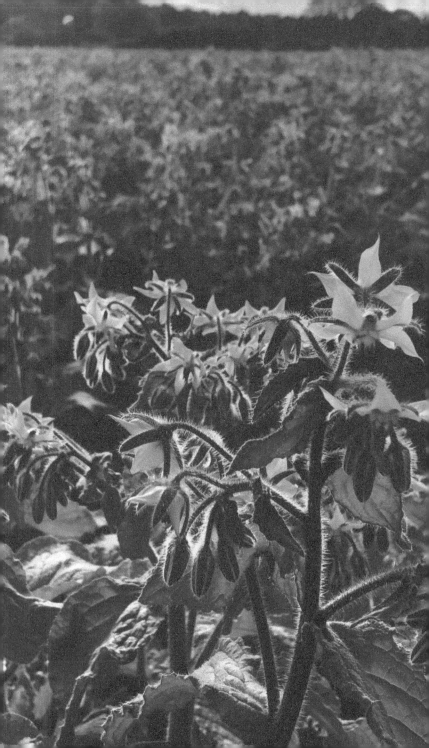

Chapter 18

B y ferry, I travelled across the short stretch of water to the North Island. There I explored beautiful Napier, with its art deco architecture, and Lake Taupo, where I attached myself to a giant of a man I'd only just met. He wore trousers with flames down the side, and we jumped out of a plane together. A last-minute decision, I had only turned up to support some fellow travellers and felt a bit worse for wear from the night before.

As we sat in the plane, I had second thoughts. My heart in my mouth, it was too late to change my mind. We skydived, and my stomach reached my mouth. My partner pulled the cord, and the chute dragged us upwards with terrific force. Then came the best bit: looking down at a miniature scene of fields and villages and houses, Lake Taupo and the mountains. It was like looking down from a plane window but more intense, and I could look in any direction. As we slowly descended, I saw the landscape as a bird might - circles of trees from just above their canopies and rivers as sparkling ribbons. I grew feathers as I swooped and whirled down to land.

I'd been invited to visit my aunt's sister, Sarah, pregnant with child number four, her strapping husband Chris and three young children. I pitched in with daily life on their dairy farm near Otorohanga and planned the rest of my trip. I hadn't seen Sarah for many years, since she emigrated, and it was unexpected that we would immediately form a natural friendship. She is a warm and welcoming soul, who quickly shepherded me into her life, treating me like one of her own and combatting any nervousness I turned up with. She spent the last baking hot weeks of her pregnancy in Canterbury rugby shorts and a bra, stomach hanging out as she entertained me with her stories, handed out jobs, and nested. They had a long driveway so she did cover up if we heard someone coming.

After being involved in a car crash, Sarah's in-laws down the road couldn't help out for a few weeks. It became clear Sarah would need some help when the baby arrived, so I extended my trip by an extra month and went off to explore, arranging to return to help when they would need it most.

I completed the Tongariro Crossing alone, walking along lunar-like, rocky paths across an extinct volcano, devoid of trees and punctuated with aquamarine pools. I wondered why I could see so many way markers, until the cloud abruptly came down. Without them, I would have been entirely lost. Coming down the side of the volcano was like encountering a sleeping dragon, with steam pouring out of cracks in the ground. Before this trip, I had never hiked anywhere alone for more than 30 minutes. I found the experience empowering and liberating.

After a trip to the East Cape and Gisborne to see Māori homesteads and the world's most easterly sunrise, I returned to Otorohanga. Living in the converted garage next to their modest house, stunning, gently rolling hills became a familiar backdrop. And cows, a lot of black-and-white Friesian-Jersey cows. I slotted into their routine, driving the children to kindergarten barefoot and waving back at everyone who drove past. I didn't have a clue who anybody was, but they all knew me. Everyone knew everyone which turned out to be helpful when my car tyre blew out. We veered all over the road, but I managed a reasonably calm emergency stop on the verge. What now? Stuck in the middle of nowhere, I wasn't sure I even knew the farm address. Little legs couldn't walk that far. A car stopped, and the driver knew who we were and where we lived by looking at our vehicle and the children. We had to trust him, and he returned us, safe and sound.

Sarah left me with the new baby whilst she went to carry out a job on the farm. She'd not left him alone before, but Kissy, the huge mastiff dog, protected him by sitting on one side of the doorway, and a small white chicken with a red comb sat on the other side. Ten minutes later, the baby started wailing and didn't stop until Sarah came back, his tiny lungs unexpectedly loud, oblivious to any effort to calm him.

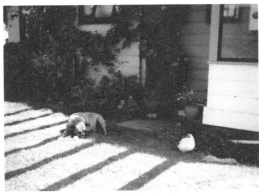

Kissy and the chicken

I fell completely fell in love with all four children, and it was tough to leave. But leave, I must. I couldn't keep putting my life on hold.

I travelled by small airplane to a hostel on a remote island. Reading in the hostel one morning, I looked up to see a young Japanese man returning from fishing. He prepared fresh sushi in front of me, the best I had ever tasted. Despite us not being able to speak each other's languages I somehow conveyed my wonder and thanks at the dish he produced.

The electricity on the island came from generators and went off at 11 p.m. We walked home from the bar each night by starlight or, if there was cloud cover, by studiously following the white lines at the edge of the road to avoid falling in the water.

Most days I hitched a ride to the beach with some surfers I'd just met and lazed on the sand, reading, paddling and beach-combing until they were ready to return. An almost perfect sea urchin and two paua, or mother-of-pearl, shells were carefully wrapped and packed to come home with me, to sit on my windowsill for decades to come. The only proof I was ever there, having taken no photos and later forgetting the name of the island and all of the people I met.

I reluctantly returned to the UK, but made a bit of a faux pas. I gave my parents the flight details but realised that I'd mixed up the dates due to different time zones. They would be coming to pick me up twenty-four hours too early. They had a two- to three-hour drive to the airport, and we'd not seen each other for seven months. I got hold of my Aunt Marion who in turn contacted Heathrow airport, and my parents heard their names over the address system. Panicking, they went to the desk to be told that I would not be coming home that day. Whoops. Deflated, they went home only to return the next day, on a much busier Monday morning. Airports are such emotional places, full of heartfelt hellos and tender goodbyes. Being reunited was very special and much nicer than leaving them all those months previously.

I returned home a different person. I'd seen nature on a whole different scale and gained some much-needed perspective. I dearly wanted to go back to New Zealand, but I had to get a job first. I wasn't in Essex for long before a friend offered me a room in London, and off I went into the big smoke. You know what happened next.

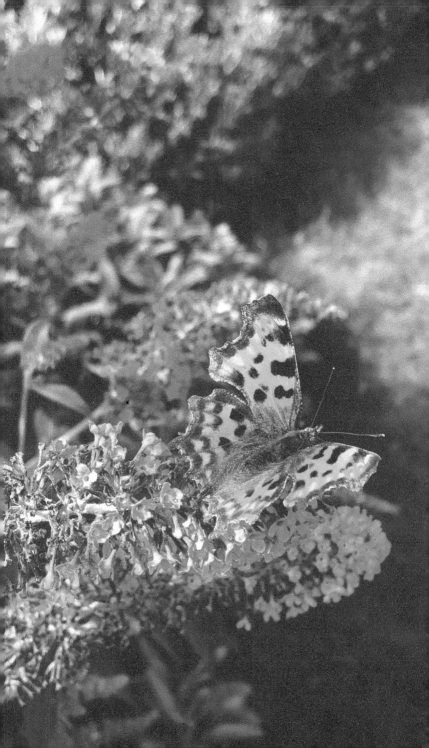

Chapter 19

Fast-forward to 2011. Within months of D's Beachy Head proposal, we had sold my maisonette and D's flat, swapping them for a detached house less than three miles from my childhood home and the garden centre in North Essex. Moving here meant we had our own garden. Living in a flat with walks and the River Thames on the doorstep certainly had its advantages, but I now found the city tiring to navigate, and the rural way of life was calling me. D and I wanted any children to be raised free-range.

We moved in July, the month Nanny Bourne died. Dad and I saw her the day before, and her memory had really deteriorated. Once a minute, every minute, she repeated the same words, 'What am I supposed to do?', and I had to leave her room to avoid showing her my distress. She had only recently moved into a care home after living in a detached house on her own for ten years; being in her eighties, she'd done very well to last so long. After she died, Dad said I could have some of her garden tools, including a ladies' fork, which is the perfect size. I use it most weeks and always think of her when I reach to pick up the well-worn wooden handle. Her hands would have been where my hands now are, and our shared love of nature still connects us. During World War II, she became a Land Girl, so even before she moved to Perrywood with Les, she really understood the value of the terrain and the meaning of hard work.

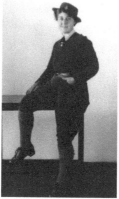

Mary (Nanny) in her Land Girl uniform

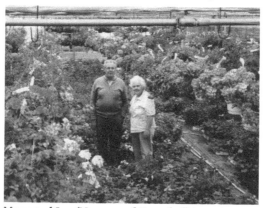

Mary and Les (Nanny and Grandad) in retirement

Two months after moving, we got married. When planning our wedding day, the flowers and the food filled my thoughts the most. I was less bothered about the dress, if I'm honest. Just as well, as the seamstress we hired to make some alterations cocked things up, although I don't think anyone else noticed. Dad brought in two silver birch trees with white trunks for the front of the ceremony room, underplanted with Perrywood-grown claret cyclamen. How perfect to have a piece of the garden centre ahead of me as I walked down the aisle with him to Pachelbel's Canon.

A good friend's brother grows natural 'garden flowers' and did us proud with bouquets, buttonholes and jars of blooms on the tables. I asked for rosemary to be included for its Mediterranean aroma, which I knew D loved. Garden flowers such as astrantia, hydrangea, roses, nigella, cotinus, with dill to help soften the flowers, setting a relaxed mood on a beautiful, sunny autumnal day. We posed for pictures amongst the horse chestnut trees, with the black Essex barn behind us and ploughed fields to the side.

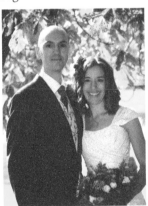

The happy couple

By now, my health had improved a lot. The twitches only occurred at osteopathy appointments, and the tremor had disappeared completely. I still got easily tired and hadn't gone back to drinking alcohol or eating wheat. Working part-time gave me space to look after myself and attend health appointments. I felt nervous leaving behind my faithful London practitioners who had been my support network. I wasn't ready to let go of their treatments altogether, though.

My osteopath recommended someone local who actually taught him in the past. Sure enough, after one appointment, I trusted her with my health. With the acupuncture, I researched online, hoped for the best and struck lucky there, too.

The Essex countryside welcomed me back with open arms, and I bored D silly as I reconnected with the wild places we loved as children. Friday Woods with its knotty, crooked trees and the scary rope swing over the stream, paths well-trodden by Colchester Garrison army troops in training. Tiptree Heath, where I once helped build piles of gorse and brambles and burned them, as community service for one of my Duke of Edinburgh awards. It's the only place in Essex where you will see all three heather species growing together and it's the county's most significant area of lowland heath. The causeway over Abberton Reservoir is a haven for birds, which often stop in the middle of the road, oblivious to any danger. This is also the way to the beaches of Mersea Island, where I am now too big to get inside the World War II pillboxes without panicking.

We made brand new memories too, falling in love with the peace and tranquillity of the Markshall Estate. It has trees from around the world, including one of the largest collections of the rare Wollemi pines outside of Australia. Less than 100 exist in the wild and they have been growing on Earth for at least 90 million years.

In London, I'd had to educate colleagues about North Essex, with its striking coastal mudflats, picturesque arable fields and ancient woodland. I carried with me the burden of being an Essex Girl, regularly batting away the prevalent '80s stigma. So, it was good to be back with those who knew the secrets Essex held.

We had an Indian summer during October, and D and I rendezvoused with family on the ten-metre-wide beach at Goldhanger's sea wall. We parked next to St Peter's, a flint church that has probably been a religious site since the Saxon times. Passing my grandparents' gravestones and ominous yew trees, we stepped over the unusual stile, a wooden Y in the brick-and-stone wall. Beyond the wheat fields, the Blackwater Estuary lay in front of us. Leaving the footpath behind, we made the short climb up onto the sea wall, built to protect the land from high tides. We wound our way around the creek, where bones of boat wrecks from my childhood still endured, the wood slow to rot. Just past the sailing club starter's hut, we reached our destination and stopped to take in the view. The majestic sailing barges from Maldon with their distinctive red sails floated in the middle of the channel, joined by a scattering of dinghies from the various sailing clubs.

My wider family met us there. Mum grew up in the village, with the sea wall as her playground. The high water lapped against stones near the steps down from the raised sea wall path. The estuary was as calm as a millpond and mirrored the waif-like wisps of cloud in the big, blue sky above. I waded in, up to my waist, and pushed myself off the warm mud into the inviting, salty water. Surely life couldn't get much better. Afterwards, we barbecued sausages and sat in our towels, munching our hot dogs whilst we finished drying off. Tired but happy, we trekked back to the car, and D agreed, it's a very special place.

At work, the Perrywood family and the business had grown somewhat. Being among people who loved plants was a balm; I didn't realise how much I'd missed being with a green-fingered tribe. I got cracking and rebranded the business with a new logo, uniform and updated adverts. At first, I needed direction, lost without a set budget and no 'to do' list set by someone else. After a while, I realised I needed to create my own role. I was no longer part of a communications team. I was the communications team. I reacquainted myself with every aspect of the company, asking questions and finding my feet. Throwing my hat entirely into the ring scared me. Continuing to work for the business, whilst keeping other clients, suited me down to the ground.

My brother Simon worked there full-time. He'd been the least likely to want to and so, of course, was the first sibling to return. After university, he went to find an alternative career, believing that running a family business was too much like hard work. Naturally, he found that all jobs were challenging and that having a boss could be even more restrictive. Simon wasn't much into plants when we were younger. He and Tristan were more interested in the building projects, the machinery and the vehicles, so it's no wonder they both became mechanical engineers. Simon now has more houseplants than me and loves plants with attractive foliage. Like many people, he found his passion for plants later in life.

D had never lived outside of a city before, the detached houses and village life were something of a culture shock. The roads were busier than he hoped for – we were in rural Essex, not Wales where he used to holiday – and apart from a bit of common land over the road, there was nowhere to walk to from the front door. Those river paths on the flat's doorstep really spoilt us.

In our new home, we had a sixty-foot back garden to play with. What's more, there were no vixens to scare me away. I had a blank canvas, and immediately set out to add lots of plants. Tentative in my first steps, I surrounded a vegetable bed with railway sleepers and created borders with much-needed greenery and texture. We are on clay soil here, often waterlogged in winter and rock hard in the summer. No planting can occur if there hasn't been any substantial rain and, living in the driest part of the UK, we can go for weeks or even months without decent rain.

Having a garden really is the only way to learn about plants. I knew many plant names and the theory, but putting it into practice has taught me so much. Every year I've added more plants, slowly taking over more lawn, which D was initially reluctant to see covered. We painted the brown shed a tasteful sage green. One or two flower pots became twenty, lovingly watered and tended. D is always on hand to dig, prune or paint whatever is needed. Like me, he enjoys feeding and watching the birds and admits that he wasn't expecting to get as much enjoyment out of the garden as he now does. The first time he saw a green woodpecker, he thought someone's pet parrot had flown into the garden, as he had never seen anything like it.

The first occasion I saw a greater spotted woodpecker on our peanut feeder filled me with a frisson of excitement greater than any social media 'Like' or retweet. I relaxed into the moment and soaked in the view. After the first sighting, we saw two or three, and they returned multiple times a day. Their distinctive looping flight and flash of red marked them out as they descended before they pecked, pecked, pecked like their life depended on it. The list of birds we spotted in our first few weeks kept growing: wrens, robins, blackbirds, tits (great, blue, coal and long-tailed), chaffinches, greenfinches. Over the first months, seasonal or more occasional visitors were added: song thrushes, buzzards, fieldfares, redwings and sparrowhawks.

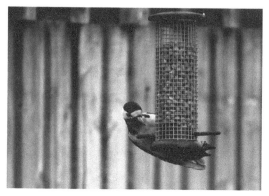

Greater Spotted Woodpecker

I'm sure our first vegetables were the best ever. Spring onions, potatoes, shallots, courgette, sweetcorn, beans, carrots, radish and beetroot. None of them perfect, and only a handful of each, but we had grown them ourselves. Herbs were plentiful: coriander, basil, rosemary, bay, thyme, parsley and mint.

I am a joiner, a member who wants to be in the gang, not left on the sidelines, which has helped my mental health over the years. There is something compelling about stumbling upon like-minded souls. Whether it's fellow bibliophiles, nature spotters, amateur artists, gardeners or writers, nothing is better than finding someone who speaks your language.

I'm lucky that my family share my excitement for nature, plants, gardening and good food. When I moved back to Essex I reconnected with good school friends, but felt an urge to further spin my web. I joined a local business networking group for women and enjoyed our monthly meetings, learning about different businesses over lunch and hearing from engaging speakers. I wanted to do something for the community so I became a school governor at a local primary school. Nativities and Year 6 leaving ceremonies were emotional affairs, and I always took a tissue.

In November, it snowed heavily. I sat in the kitchen, looking at the blanket over our garden, and marvelled at the bright, blue-white light. I saw something unusual in my peripheral vision. The conifer tree in my neighbour's garden is as tall as our house and I looked again at a shape in its branches. 'It's an owl. I think there's an owl in the tree!' Excitement fizzed through me, I couldn't believe it. I looked again through my trusty compact binoculars, and sure enough, an owl with orange eyes stared back. Excitement spilled out of me in gasps and skips, much to the amusement of D and our visiting friend, who also enjoyed the moment. Outside, I took pictures from a distance. Once we'd all had a good look, I crept even closer. The statue-still bird allowed me to get within two metres of the tree base, and I took some fantastic close-up shots. I still couldn't believe it; the bird just sat in the tree looking at me, its alert eyes unblinking. Looking it up in the book, I confirmed it was a short-eared owl that often comes out in the daytime. Honestly, this made my week, my month, possibly my year (wedding aside). We have never seen one since, so it's a once-a-decade experience so far!

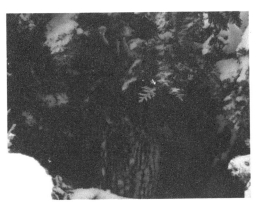

The short-eared owl

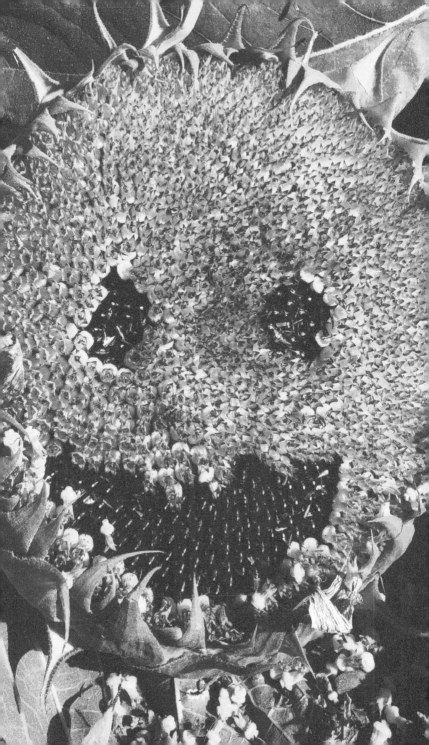

Chapter 20

When we returned from our honeymoon in March, I told my acupuncturist we were trying for a baby. She specialised in fertility acupuncture and whether by luck, her assistance or a fair wind, in the second month, I fell pregnant.

It felt like pregnancy had reset my health. I had spot-free skin, thick and glossy hair, and only mild nausea in the first few weeks. D and I took a day trip to the 2012 Olympic Games, me showing off a tiny baby bump. On our way to the basketball in the Olympic Park we became part of the unique atmosphere, everyone smiling and happy to be there. I would have been content just to visit for the planting combinations.

The banks were adorned with white and pale pink wildflowers, meadows beaming with blue cornflowers and bright yellow daisy-shaped blooms.

Trees were surrounded by sunny orange calendula. Leaving, we passed another bank planted with blue agapanthus, pink bells of dierama, yellow kniphofia (known as red-hot poker, but these ones were not red), pink diascia and a whole host of colours and flower shapes. My heart sang with joy.

My own experimental wildflower meadow was not quite up to the standard of the Olympic Park efforts but at least it

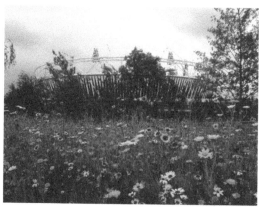

The Olympic Park

had a few flowers. More beans and lettuce were ready in the veg patch, and the onions and sweetcorn were growing at a rate of knots. I needed to do some serious weeding before planting Christmas potatoes and brassica crops to take us through the winter. Any gaps could be filled with herbs or flowers to make the most of the space.

Now thirty weeks (seven months) into my pregnancy, I enjoyed the baby kicking and moving. I never got bored of being nudged by a foot, hand or head, and I giggled when I saw the bump shaking about as the baby had a gymnastics session. I started visualising a little person, one with some kind of personality. It was extraordinary. And D could now feel the baby moving and begin to form some kind of relationship with him or her.

There were, of course, days when I felt rubbish – mentally or physically – and when I'd simply had enough. Ice packs became essential when, one weekend, the stifling summer heat gave me a rash all over my taut tummy. I wanted to scrape my nails over and over the skin, but I pulled my hands away, knowing it could make it worse. At night I couldn't sleep but draping my tummy with a cool cloth and gently moving the ice pack across gave me some relief. In the daytime a tree shaded me, nature's parasol, as I took the weight off my swollen ankles.

Physiotherapy was a lifesaver when I developed sciatica. The treatment table had a big hole in it for baby-filled bellies. After manipulation of my hip, I could again walk freely without searing, shooting pain speeding down my right leg.

Sometimes the hormones and the thought of being a mum completely overwhelmed me. There were a million decisions to be made about buggies and beds and antenatal classes and, and, and. These bad days were thankfully much rarer than the good days, and I adjusted my lifestyle to suit the pregnancy. I worked fewer hours, and tried to relax more and say no. I found it pretty challenging, and it took me a while to accept I needed to slow down. Once I did, my mindset changed. I really looked forward to giving up work altogether and hoped I'd get a few weeks of relaxation and pampering before the baby decided to arrive.

My gardening jobs continued throughout the autumn, being careful not to overbalance as I stretched down to pull up rogue weeds. The self-sufficient winter garden gave me a green view from the window, distracting me from occasional negative thoughts.

Just five days away from my due date and I was very ready to have this baby. We were organised in a practical sense and had done all the mental preparation. I experienced some Braxton Hicks (practice contractions) only to be disappointed when they weren't the real thing. I knew I had to be patient – not my strong point – and accepted that the baby would come when it was ready. Until then, I continued with my days of napping, endless snacking (I no longer had room for proper meals), reading and doing my best to stay active. I found it hard to follow the advice from friends and family of making the most of the peace and quiet we currently had when I just wanted to meet our baby.

Wanting a home birth, we hired a birthing pool and kept it running so I could get in and out as much as I liked, taking the weight off my huge tummy and easing my tight muscles. Definitely a wise investment compared to the inflatable pools, which you only put up once you are in labour.

I'd been able to switch off work within days of finishing. Work had defined me for the last fifteen years or so and been a massive part of my life. Having been forced to give it up when ill, this time I'd chosen this situation. I did miss the mental challenges. Still, it was a relief not to worry about anything else apart from myself for a change. After all, when the baby arrived, I would have to focus on someone else ...

Mid-January 2013. Light snow dusted the ground, and this week we'd discussed what would happen if it snowed more heavily and the midwife couldn't get to our house, or if we couldn't get to the hospital in an emergency. Dad wasn't far away with his 4WD and off-roading experience, if needed.

My waters broke at 3.30 a.m., and D told me to go back to sleep. After twenty minutes, I woke him again. This baby was definitely coming. D had the presence of mind to prepare for a calmer time ahead and took a homemade chocolate cake out of the freezer.

Later on, I grabbed and squeezed an inflatable gym ball and a pillow to find a way through the contractions. D's hand tried to soothe me.

'Don't touch me,' I screamed. He backed away. The birthing plan, aromatherapy, music and breathing exercises were cast aside as the waves of pain progressed quickly.

We called the midwife and expected her to be with us within twenty minutes, as the hospital is only a few miles away. She didn't turn up for ages, and we started to think we would have to deliver the baby without her.

Our calm midwife eventually arrived when the need to push was overwhelming. I could already feel the head, so she quickly got me in the pool. After more urgent pushing and some inhuman guttural wails, my daughter came out at around 8.30 a.m.

'Oh!' I exclaimed. After months of preparation, and hours of labour, I was still surprised that a baby had come out of me. There was a very short umbilical cord between us and the placenta didn't want to come out, so I got an injection in my arm, and the cord was cut sooner than planned. Too tired to detect any concern I was only vaguely aware of Daddy enjoying his first cuddle.

After a breakfast of chocolate cake, the first midwife claimed her eyesight too poor for what came next, so the 'super stitcher' midwife arrived. Lying on the living room floor for her, I looked to my side and watched in wonder. Baby E Powell (7lb 12oz) was asleep in the midwife's weighing scales.

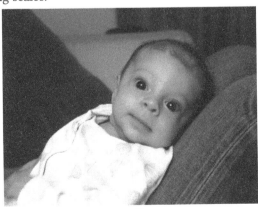

E

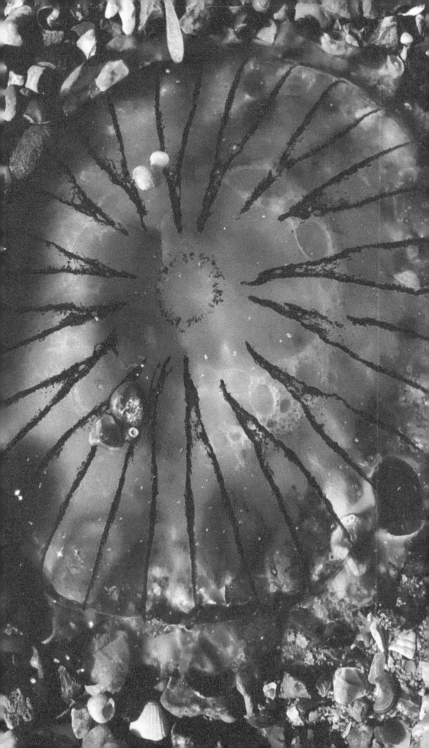

Chapter 21

For the next eight months, I rarely slept for more than an hour at a time. We neglected everything else whilst we used all our energy to keep sane and hold our lives – just about – together. Exhaustion hit every day, and the GP told me I was in danger of developing chronic fatigue syndrome. D worked in London full-time; he made snacks for me before he left for the day and lent his support the minute he got in. Sleep eluded me. The garden had been abruptly neglected. I spent my days and nights in a fog, desperately holding on to small wonders around me. Waxwings flew in and out of the garden, snatching pink sorbus berries before they disappeared for another year. The snowdrops emerged from the cold hard ground and gave me hope, each flower delicate and perfect. Pure white like a new pair of trainers, with a splash of green to give them attitude, they brought cheer when we needed it most. The sap would soon be rising.

Three months in, and my life had been completely consumed by my new daughter. There was much to recommend it. I loved everything about her. The grip of her tiny fingers and her eyes looking at me. The cuddles and smiles, especially that first smile after waking and seeing me, a gummy grin from ear to ear lighting up her face. Seeing D with her and knowing how much love she had from her wider family and us. Watching her grow and begin to explore her world. Meeting other mums and sharing highs and lows, tears and tantrums. Feeling her relax and drop off in her sling whilst I made dinner, or walked around the garden. Forgetting about work for a bit. Learning to trust my instincts as a mum and finding patience I never knew I had.

On the other side of the coin, the lack of sleep was truly torture and made everything a hundred times harder. We trudged through a minefield of conflicting information, much of it not making any sense for our baby. We heard how other babies slept for many hours when ours didn't. And the intensity of breastfeeding. As part of our antenatal class, we attended a session about feeding. They didn't tell us how difficult it could be to get to grips with it in the first place. Had I not been pig-headed, I would have given up. Eventually, she loved feeds, and wanted one every hour, so she slept in my bed next to me, leaving D in the spare room so he could get enough sleep to function at work.

The good days eventually outweighed the bad, and we found our rhythm. It could only get better. Whilst tired, I hadn't experienced any other FND symptoms. My recovery had been sustained, even when faced with extra physical and mental challenges.

Though I was not yet back at work, my days were surprisingly full, and my brain struggled to keep up. Play dates, toddler groups, mum-and-baby yoga classes. On one typical morning I got up early to go to a buggy fitness class. I then realised the buggy wheels were in D's car, and he had driven to the station with them. I drove to get them (with E screaming in the back), before rushing to class and arriving late (E now asleep), only to find the class not running. I somehow missed the memo. I felt like I'd done a day's work by only 10.17 a.m. Thankfully, E remained asleep as I took some deep breaths and reconsidered my morning plans – the silence golden.

As E learned to walk and slept better, we slowly emerged back into life as a butterfly from a chrysalis. The garden became a playground and a place to learn about wildlife. She'd totter around and want to hold the watering can and the trowel, just like Mummy. We planted seeds, grew vegetables, and I told her the names of all the plants. It melted my heart to see her enjoying nature. It wasn't just a fun activity; it's part of her heritage and it's in her blood.

A friend hired a professional nanny when she went back to work, which opened my eyes to the possibility that we could employ someone to look after our child in our home. Just before E turned one, a lovely lady, Jan, came to regularly look after her, allowing me to return to work one or two days a week and have a break from being Mum.

Though I wanted to return to my job, my identity had changed, become wholly subsumed by being a mum, and my confidence had been shaken. I wondered if I could still do it. Could I hold a normal conversation anymore? Did I have enough energy, and had I missed too much? How would E cope?

Hiring a nanny turned out to be the best decision ever. Not only did E completely adore being with Jan, but while E slept or played, she cooked a meal, tidied or did some washing. What's more, she had a granddaughter the same age, so E had a better social life than I did, going on play dates and visits to farms, playgrounds and zoos.

It took about three months to believe in myself again at work and to fire up the part of my brain which could converse with adults and make sense of the garden centre world. Having a break from E meant when I spent time with her, I could be much more patient, and a better mum.

I would have liked more children. Having two siblings and spending a lot of time with three younger cousins growing up, I never envisaged only having one. But my health only just survived the experience of having a baby, and reluctantly D and I agreed that it was best to stick with our one beautiful, special girl. The idea of doing it all again with a toddler in tow didn't appeal. I grieve for the siblings she will never have. I can't imagine not having my two brothers, but being an only child will be normal for her.

A friend made me feel better by saying that many women are broody and sad after they stop having babies, whether they stop at just one or go on to have three or four.

There is always an expectation that a second child will follow, and people couldn't help but ask, even those who didn't know me very well. When they did ask, I'd joke and say, 'No, one was enough.' They meant well, but it did leave me feeling sad.

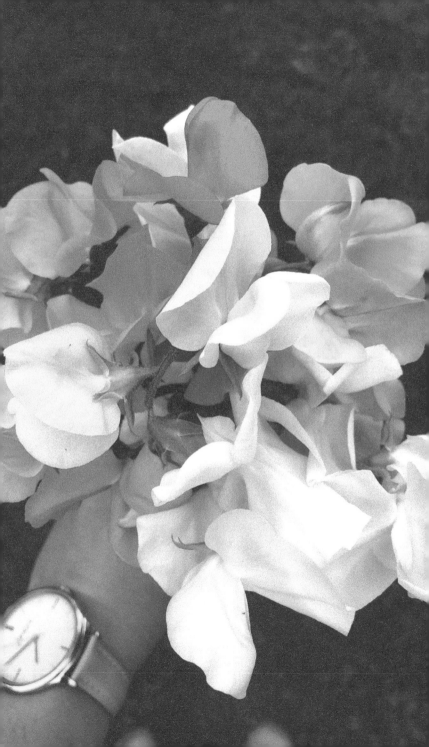

Chapter 22

O ur first holidays with a child were wonderful but such hard work. Whilst packing all the paraphernalia we wondered if it was worth the effort. The year E turned one, things seemed to get easier, so we went a bit further afield and drove to the Peak District in May. E cried for most of the journey. We arrived on edge, tired and irritable, to a welcoming stone house on the edge of the national park, surrounded by fields of hardy sheep, crumbling dry stone walls and hills we would love to climb in the distance.

The nights were dreadful. E was teething and simply didn't want to sleep without one of us next to her. The daylight soothed our fractious minds and we enjoyed sunny spring days watching lambs frolic and visiting stately home gardens full of loud, bright azaleas, rhododendrons and yellow laburnum. This was what I would take home with me.

In September we met up with Portsmouth friends. D's best man, also our first date chaperone, and his family had been sorely neglected whilst we tended to our baby and focused on surviving. E had her first paddle in the sea and we enjoyed reconnecting.

We spent the rest of the week in another holiday house in the New Forest; thankfully, we all got more sleep this time. More gardens to visit, featuring pink spiky dahlias and swathes of yellow rudbeckia, daisy-shaped with brown centres. Kitchen gardens full of rainbow chard with dark green leaves and yellow, red and white candy-like stems. Green and purple basil that made us hungry for pizza as we brushed against it. Treehouses and fairy doors. Everywhere an adventure, seen through a one-year-old's eyes. I was in my element.

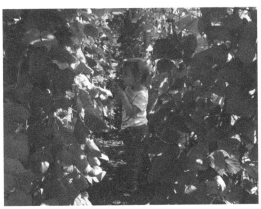

In the bean arches – New Forest

May 2015, Sussex. The formula of holidaying in an area where our abandoned friends lived was, again, a huge success. There in May for bluebell season, we got the children and families to pose for pictures. I had made these friends in London when life was hectic and selfish, and here we were, three children between us, relaxing in a wood full of bluebells. The contrast was striking, yet we still had much in common.

In Sheffield Park, a professional photographer approached us. 'Can I take a picture of your daughter running to you in front of the bright pink azalea bushes?' We posed and laughed and wondered if the photos would be in the papers. They weren't, but he kindly sent us copies.

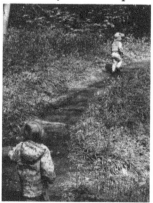

In the bluebells

In our rented holiday house, we investigated the old magnolia tree in the garden, branches covered in grey and orange lichen. It was a joy to point out these wonders to our daughter, whose personality was developing. Stubborn and strong-willed, curious about the world around her. Each day she chose her own clothes, which were bright and perfectly mismatched. I taught both E and D to stop and notice the natural world around them, just like Nanny, Mum and Dad did with me. There is something wondrous about observing small details that may have been missed by others, serving to slow life down, bring colour and interest to our lives, and I enjoyed passing on a skill which would perhaps help E with her mental health in the future.

On our return, we reflected that we could be more adventurous now. Little legs were getting more robust, and sleeping in strange beds was at least possible, if not guaranteed. As soon as we got home, I started the process of researching and booking our next trip.

We packed in the holidays before E started school. In September 2016, we headed to the south west coast of France. Just being there energised me; it was a textural feast for the senses. Lines of white and grey breakers crashed onto the long, golden beach, entrancing us but never calming down enough for us to swim. Tractors carved lines in the sand, in contrast to the smoothness around them. I loved the edges and shadows they created, changing as the sun moved through the sky then started to disappear over the water. Footsteps made more dynamic lines, randomly scattered as if someone had thrown stones up in the air to make marks where they fell. Pine trees scented the air, reminding me of my Danish adventures, casting silhouettes across the darkening sky. On the beach and back in our garden for the week, we sorted, gathered – and sometimes discarded – gigantic, rough fir cones, smooth pink and white pebbles, shells of every colour and water-worn driftwood. An enormous moth enthralled us with its soft, hairy, wood-effect wings and flashes of dark red on its body.

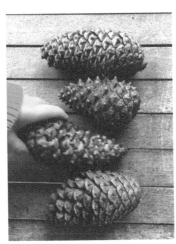

Collecting pine cones

There at the end of the season, the French were nonchalant about opening restaurants. It was pot luck whether we could find something to eat or not. Walking around Bayonne, hoping we would find more going on, we'd look up to see which vines or vegetables were growing on the townhouse balconies. We spotted spiky agave leaves poking out from a rooftop garden. Having sought out busy streets, we found ourselves seeking a moment of calm, finding it in a botanic garden where we watched orange-and-white koi carp lazily circling their pool.

Closer to home, and in between the booked holidays, there was much to enjoy. We often took the short journey to Suffolk, one of our childhood haunts, and a favourite for day trips. In my teens, my parents bought a place to escape to, and now a third generation enjoyed exploring here. When we arrived at the bungalow, we'd stop and caress the soft, billowing grasses and the fragrant lavender bushes which led to the door. In the peaceful village where Mum and Dad spent days away from the busy garden centre, we'd watch the wind blowing across ripening barley and straw bales being stacked higher than felt safe. We'd walk from their back garden to the park where we played cricket, and from the front garden to the friendly local pub where Dad played in the boules team and sampled local ales. We'd draw faces on stones on the beach, competing to find the funniest features, each person believing theirs was the winner. We beachcombed up and down the coast and agreed that Sizewell, despite being under the watchful gaze of the power station, was one of our favourite haunts. There, the weather-worn black wooden huts charmed us, along with colourful boats and piles of fishing paraphernalia, wild flowers down to the beach and a rusting metal structure in the sea housing hundreds of noisy seabirds. On hot days we swam there, wriggling in and out of our swimming things behind towels. On one very special day we even saw a lone porpoise swimming in the waves.

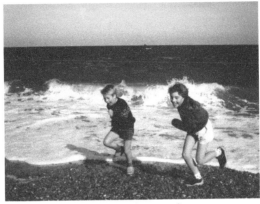

Simon and Hannah

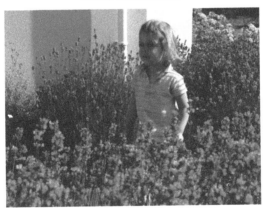

The lavender path

We'd journey down winding roads to Captain's Wood to see the ancient, gnarled oaks and the bluebells. A cold, salty wind blew across fields from the coast, meaning flowers were slow to come out here. Sometimes we'd go too early in the year, the ground yet to be smudged with blue.

We'd go in kayaks, canoes, rowing boats and motorised boats with tour guides. We'd eat from the Suffolk larder repeatedly, enjoying dressed crab, muntjac vindaloo, new potatoes and asparagus, Sutton Hoo chicken and Blythburgh pork. The pigs out in the fields had a good life. Every visit, we'd go to Aldeburgh, with its stony beach and charming high street. It was worth queuing for fish and chips, which we'd eat sitting on a concrete wall looking out to sea, whilst screeching gulls wheeled around and swooped in to snatch discarded chips. Later, we'd debate which of the many ice cream shops to frequent, and inevitably settle on Harris & James with its mouth-watering homemade ice cream and chocolate.

Suffolk is home from home, and perfectly peaceful. I breathe deeper, walk slower and drink in any up-close-and-personal encounters with the flora and fauna. Deer meander through pink and purple heather, hares box amongst the barley stubble and owls ghost silently across fertile fields, looking for their next meal. We are happy to lose track of time here, it has become a refuge when any of us need to recharge and unwind.

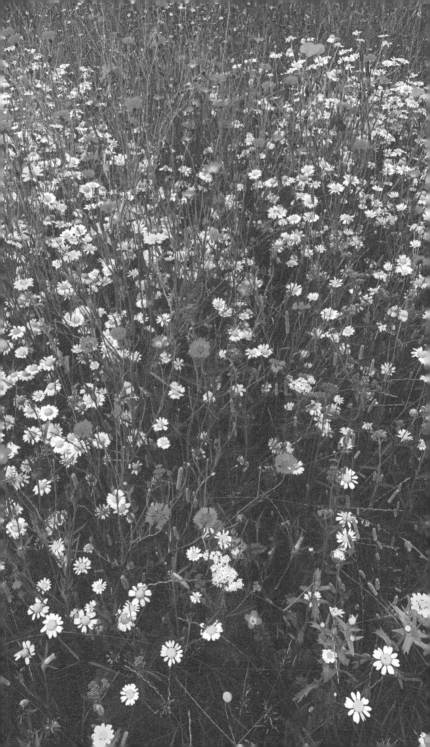

Chapter 23

2017

With E at preschool, the garden projects began again in earnest. With the back garden now well established, only the veg garden and the many pots needed our annual attention.

My gaze fell onto the front garden, an unexciting twenty-by ten-metre lawn which we never used. We needed a relaxing planting scheme to soothe us and to become a habitat for insects and birds. I had heard about the Charles Dowding 'no dig' approach and decided to give it a go.

We covered the entire lawn in large, flattened cardboard boxes from work and dampened them down with a hose. I ordered garden waste mulch from the local compost facility. The farmer who tipped the eight tonnes of compost onto the cardboard responded doubtfully to my idea, and my dad thought I was mad, too. That generation tended to rely on weedkillers or machinery to get rid of turf. We had to spread out the mulch one shovel or rake full at a time, and I found muscles I never knew I had. I added hard-to-shift heavy topsoil to give the soil a better texture and more nutrients, biting off more than I could chew. We asked our neighbour's son to come and help finish the job, which was much appreciated.

The cardboard rotted down and, after a few weeks, the grass underneath died, leaving us with lovely compost to plant into. We planted perennials easily into the soft top layer. When we had to dig deeper into the clay for trees and shrubs it became more difficult. As we dug, there were no cardboard boxes to be found, only pieces of tape. The rotted cardboard added helpful carbon, and I went to bed relieved that my plan was working.

Seeking calm and tranquillity, I chose a palette of blue, white, pale yellow and acid green. This was a departure from my go-to colours in the back garden – purple and yellow – a scheme which developed accidentally because of the plants which sung to me, and found themselves in my trolley. Initially sure of my planting scheme on paper, there were many changes as I laid the plants out and discovered my mistakes. I gained a new-found respect for the garden designers winning gold medals at the RHS Chelsea Flower Show each year.

The garden brings us great joy and we stop and look often. A few perennial weeds have persisted, but most weeds and all the grass were killed by the cardboard. I considered what this project had taught me so far. The no-dig cardboard method was effective – but not easy. I over-ambitiously took on quite a large space, but I would do it again in smaller areas or in stages. It works particularly well on top of clay soils, which can be hard to dig once they dry out.

Mulching annually keeps down weeds and retains moisture. Each spring, I add more mulch, organic matter for the worms to take down into the clay soil, and to retain as much moisture as possible.

All flower beds benefit from some structure and height. For my garden, I used a mix of gravel, bark and corten steel edging, together with a birch tree, evergreen shrubs - including winter box (sarcococca) - and small dwarf pines. My oversized black pot also provides a focal point. I varied the foliage types – mixing grasses with larger leaves on hostas and alchemilla mollis. The mix of flowers has attracted lots of pollinators. Flowering hellebores, pulmonaria and bulbs like crocus and camassia help insects with an early nectar source. If you want a natural-looking garden, scattering seed from self-seeding plants, like foxgloves and love-in-a-mist, will give you many more in the years that follow.

As I weeded in my new paradise one afternoon, the farmer who dropped off the compost drove past in his tractor. I waved, hoping he enjoyed his bird's-eye view and wondering whether he had changed his mind about my mad methods. Dad liked the space I created, and my colour combinations, but I knew he would always prefer to use a digger to create a new flower bed. Mum told me my planting wouldn't be out of place in Kew Gardens.

It's a beautiful place to wait for my daughter's school bus in the mornings, like opening the pages of our very own Secret Garden. There are many insects, and we have left a wild patch in the corner with nettles and weeds to encourage them to visit. The annual mulch is very popular with the rose chafer beetle, which we had never seen in the garden before planting it up. I uncover larvae each time I dig, and in the summer, to our delight, the show-stopping, emerald-green beetles take flight and buzz around us like metallic clockwork toys. The boring lawn has metamorphosed from a drawing and a pile of soil into a medley of colours, textures and uplifting experiences.

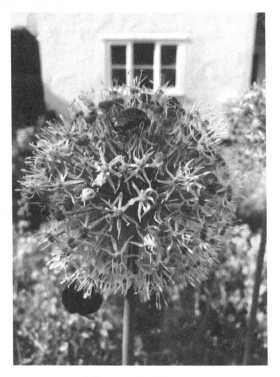

Allium and pollinators

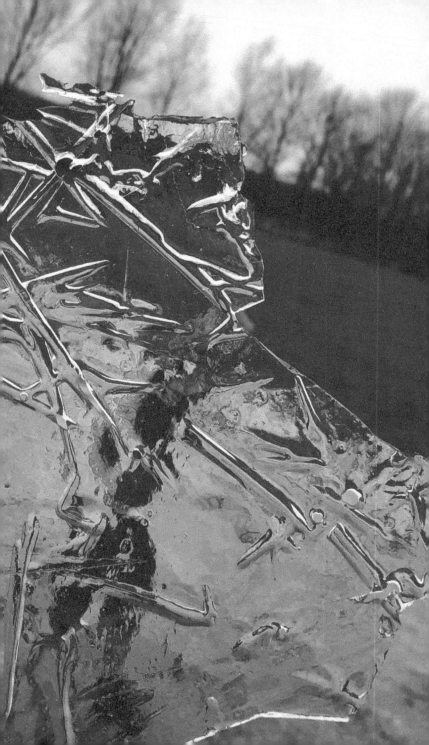

Chapter 24

P errywood ran parallel to all my own gardening and life events and the garden centre grew from strength to strength.

I sat in the audience overawed at my first Garden Centre Association (GCA) Conference, daunted to meet the owners of some of the most successful, award-winning garden centres in the UK and motivated to get some of the accolades for ourselves.

After becoming members, we entered the top 100 league table of UK garden centres at 75. We learned what they were looking for and went up to 25. The team and our customers were delighted.

Well, imagine our pleasure, and disbelief, if I'm honest, when we kept improving, dipping into the teens and the top ten. Then in 2018 we were named fourth-best garden centre in the UK. The champagne flowed that night, once we'd picked our jaws up off the floor. Our hard work and continuous improvement was paying off. We placed third again the next year, and again in 2020. We now had our eyes on the number one and number two slots, but the competition was fierce.

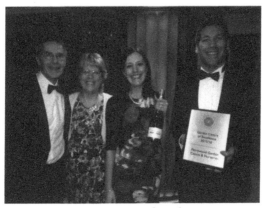

Alan, Karin, Hannah and Simon

Running alongside the award for best garden centre was an equally intense competition for best fancy dress. We perhaps took our business value of 'being the best you can be' a bit far. From matching golf outfits in St Andrews, to pop stars in Brighton. At last, dressed as gnomes from Gnomeo & Juliet in Stratford - a slightly left-field take on a Shakespeare theme - we gained a top three place.

The owners I was so daunted by were open and generous with their time and encouragement, and became friends. We joined their ranks, with pictures of our garden centre featuring on the big screen to inspire others.

Conference speakers left a lasting legacy. Keynote and business coach Michael Heppell told us how to be brilliant, and has since helped me to write this book. Ex-BBC HR Director Lucy Adams persuaded us to ditch appraisals, which no one misses. Retail expert Ken Hughes encouraged us to try something new every day, which in turn led me to do forty challenges for my fortieth birthday. My varied tasks included hula-hooping, performing a rap dance (cringe), turning off my phone for a week, making sushi, writing and illustrating a children's book and hitting a golf ball 100 yards. No bras were involved this time and I raised more than £1,000 for my local branch of MIND. I had hoped to finish before my big birthday. It took a lot longer, and I didn't have the energy to speed things up, so I gave myself a break and extended the finish line into my forty-first year.

Tristan now joined the Perrywood team. When he joined as a contractor, he got stuck in, managing the build of a new staffroom and coffee-shop kitchen extension. Like me, he loved being part of our family team, and joined us full-time. The team continued to grow, and we were now responsible for a much bigger family of 175. We were big enough to have a communications team, which took over the day-to-day marketing efforts. I love having their creative brains around me, and their friendship.

Finding I had time to spare, I took on responsibility for HR, wanting to improve the way we supported the team and to help them with their well-being in the workplace.

One of the things I love most about running a business is the opportunity to visit other gardens and garden centres, all in the name of work. Staying in London for the wedding of a family friend, Mum, Dad and I visited The Chelsea Gardener, a small, expensive garden centre, which was just the kind of place you'd expect to bump into an A-list celebrity. As I looked around their shop, I saw someone I knew, but where from? From Four Weddings and a Funeral and numerous other films and interviews, that's where from.

Hugh Grant stood in front of Mum and me with his family. We tried to act nonchalantly, allowing ourselves surreptitious glances. I tried out an uber-cool inflatable garden chair, trusting it with all my weight, before it flew to one side and I landed directly on the hard floor beneath. Whoops. I let out a screech and a laugh and I realised it looked like I was trying to get Hugh Grant's attention, hoping he would come to my aid. He didn't. Instead, Dad appeared and pulled me up, and Hugh walked the other way, saying to his wife, 'Let's go and look for some pots.'

Mum retired due to ill health, leaving Dad, myself, and 'the boys' in charge. In board meetings, we discussed how we were reaching the limits of what we could do at Perrywood Tiptree. We were ambitious and wanted to buy another garden centre. In 2018, Wyevale put its 120 garden centres on the market. We visited those in Essex, Suffolk and even in Norfolk. We wanted to buy one but put in bids for several in the hope of attracting the vendors' notice. It worked, and several months after they went up for sale, we got the keys to their Sudbury branch, in Suffolk. First came a period of secrecy under the terms of a non-disclosure agreement. Only trusted advisors and immediate family knew about it. We squirrelled ourselves away to go through all the due diligence and prepare for the next phase. I worked evenings and weekends to get it all done, getting tired, but I couldn't afford to stop. We were nearly there and a two week holiday in Denmark revived me. I felt exhausted but had enough energy to meet up with family and friends, revisiting childhood haunts and creating new memories with D and E. Now five, she wanted more from her holidays. This time when we went to the Djurs Sommerland theme park, we avoided the water rafting ride that Tristan cracked his head on all those years ago. E enjoyed the safer rides and declared this the 'best day ever.'

At work, I worried that we'd taken on too much. Imposter syndrome nibbled away at me, making me question whether I could do this or not. We gathered the Tiptree team in the coffee shop one morning. They looked at us expectantly, and some of them wondered if Dad would be retiring. We announced that we had bought a new garden centre and they burst into applause. I realised I had been holding my breath. We'd been talking about this for months in a bubble, and we didn't know how they would react. Getting their support was crucial to the next stage.

We drove to Sudbury to introduce ourselves as the new owners. A swarm of eels jiggled around in my stomach, making me feel sick. My nerves were jangling. Thankfully, as a family business that wanted to keep the garden centre running, we were well-received. We went for a family lunch to celebrate, but I struggled to eat anything, my stomach now blown up like I was eight months pregnant.

In the two years since the purchase, I have grown used to running two centres; we hired an HR manager to take on the day-to-day work and address the team's concerns, which has made an enormous difference both to our staff's well-being and to my own mental health. It's made it easier for me to take a step back when my health demands it, and when I do need to step into a project, I have the energy to do so. I've been fortunate to be able to design my role around what I like doing and what I can do.

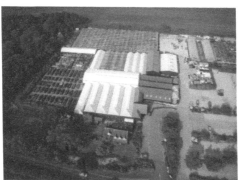

Perrywood Tiptree - 2014

Chapter 25

It is drummed into us that we must exercise to be healthy. In primary school and into my teens I was part of a netball team, but I would certainly never describe myself as sporty. I once came third in the school cross-country run, but with only four in the race (and one who dropped out halfway), it was hardly a victory, particularly because I was competing at the same time as the runners from the year below, who all beat me too. Even my own brother, Simon, heckled me on the finish line for my pathetic performance.

Since being ill I have gone back to both yoga and Pilates, supposedly gentle, but neither worked for me this time. They caused soft tissue injuries and I spent too much time and money on osteopathy to fix the subsequent damage. My body is not the same as it once was, and I had to downgrade my expectations.

Instead, tai chi, with its slow, purposeful movements, became a weekly meditation. On joining, I brought down the average age in the class by considerable years, but I didn't care. We had a common goal: to improve our health, and I found it to be very grounding. It settled me back into myself and calmed the ongoing internal twitchiness of my nervous system, invisible to others. Outsiders may have watched us creating circles with our hands and arms and thought we weren't doing a lot but, inside, our bodies were working hard. I often headed home exhausted, in part because of the exercises but also, in slowing down, I realised how worn out I was.

By 2019, appointments with my cranial osteopath stopped, unneeded, and I reduced the acupuncture from monthly to every six-to-eight weeks, or more. Since living in Essex, I've seen a couple of nutritionists in another effort to beat regular fatigue and to help with irritable bowel syndrome. The nutritionists also supported me when I picked up a Helicobacter pylori infection, which affected my stomach lining and caused heartburn. I reluctantly took antibiotics to kill the harmful bacteria that caused the problems. It killed the healthy gut flora too, so later I took supplements to boost their levels.

Swimming let me increase my heart rate without putting pressure on my joints and soft tissues. I'd ache the next day but my muscles quickly recovered. I've reverted to walking each week, which is good as long as I don't walk too far or too fast. After a two-and-a-half-hour brisk walk and talk with a friend, I was in agony for two weeks, although I was trying to skip every day for charity at the time, which probably didn't help. The skipping only lasted a few days before I gave up in pain.

In September I became breathless after getting a cold and got an inhaler from the asthma nurse. Mum developed late-onset asthma, so it could have been that. For a different reason, I got some blood tests done, and my GP told me a rare genetic condition had been flagged which needed investigating. They were not sure why I had been screened for this; the doctor must have ticked the wrong box on the blood test form. My thoughts became darker as I thought about what this meant, and my mental health concerned me. I returned to counselling to stop this decline and ensure it didn't descend too far. Eventually, the doctor told me it wasn't a worrying kind of genetic condition unless I smoked. All that worry around a test I should never have had in the first place.

As we entered the Covid-19 pandemic, my anxieties understandably increased. I found it hard going from keeping 200 team members physically and mentally safe, with stringent guidelines in place, to other environments where I couldn't control events. I shied away from others in public places and even found it weird watching TV programmes filmed pre-Covid-19 where people looked too close together. Counselling sessions took on a new meaning and kept me from overly worrying about the events that were unfolding, and what might happen to me and those I loved.

Filled to overflowing with varying emotions, it was hard to process them some days. Closing our business for six weeks was difficult. Never before had I experienced such uncertainty. Two weeks into the lockdown we started offering local deliveries. With most of my team furloughed, I updated our weekly availability lists by going to the garden centre once a week to take photos of plants and getting the information uploaded to the website. This may sound fairly easy, but I felt a lot of pressure to get it done quickly and accurately, especially as we didn't know how long it would go on for.

Outside of work, the lockdowns allowed me to explore nature's local haunts with D and E. Told by Prime Minister

Boris not to travel too far, we often went to Pitts Wood in Copford, Layer Woods, and the Causeway at Abberton Reservoir, and we walked for miles along the footpaths in Layer Marney and Layer de la Haye. We experienced the changing seasons through a narrowed lens. Blinkered like horses we noticed more, picking up on glorious changes as spring sprung.

On one of our early walks, we did a loop round Layer Marney Tower and gazed at the tall, red-brick Tudor palace, giddy at the thought of having such a wonderful building on our doorstep.

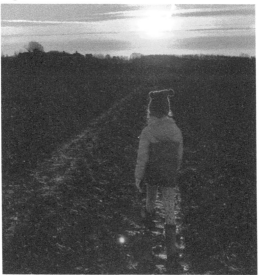

The footpath to Layer Marney Tower

At home, the three of us were struggling with enforced captivity. We took a while to adjust to being in such close proximity. We snapped and snarled as we drew boundaries around ourselves and argued about who could use the inadequate broadband. E understandably grieved at the temporary loss of her best friend, and desperately missed playing with other children. She tried to control what little freedom she had been left with. She didn't want to do her schoolwork. She didn't want to go outside. It would take arguments and bribes to get her in the car, but it was worth the effort to see her skipping ahead of us later on. After twenty minutes, sometimes more, she relaxed in the outdoors and we caught a glimpse of the girl she used to be. We walked two dogs for a friendly neighbour, using them as another reason to get out of the house. The Border collie was calmer than my Tilly used to be, but when we threw a ball for her, boy, she really motored. Our smiles broadened and E squealed in delight.

In lockdown one, the woods were still bare, and we startled woodcock (or snipe) from their hiding places, recognising them by their long beaks and zigzag flight. In ten years, we'd never seen them before. Lichens and mosses held our gaze, almost glowing to catch our attention in their dull brown surroundings. Slowly, things came to life. Canopies of leaves gradually hid the sky, unfolding one by one to start with, then seemingly all at once in the sunshine. Leaf mould gave life to growth on the ground, ferns unfurling to reveal their regal stature. Catkins puffed out pollen and cuckoo song marked the start of spring.

In our garden we found pleasure in planting, weeding, bug hunting, and just sitting and letting the sun soak in.

Suddenly, it all clicked into place. I spent most of my childhood on the same patch of land, trod the same paths daily when ill and, lastly, revisited the same walks and woods during lockdown. Each time, I was forced to look closer, breathe deeper and cherish simple pleasures. In childhood it was just being, I didn't know it wasn't what everyone else did. As an adult, this process of reduction soothed me during chaotic times. Twice, it healed me.

We lost my mother-in-law, Dorothy, to the coronavirus during April. She was in her eighties with emphysema, so the virus quickly took hold. Not being able to go and see her was incredibly cruel for the family. She died in hospital and, during her two weeks there, she wasn't allowed to receive any visitors.

I often think about her as I garden. She grew up in Carmarthen, Wales, where her dad (a tailor) had an allotment and her auntie a farm. For someone who lived all her adult life in the suburbs of Great Barr, Birmingham, she was very in tune with the seasons and the natural world and tended a modest garden. She loved bright flowers and enjoyed looking around our plot when she visited. As she grew older, she lived in the past, and conversations would invariably lead to her saying, 'my mum used to grow that' or 'my dad used to have those on his allotment.'

Only D went back for the funeral, a sad affair attended by her two loving sons. We hope for the day we can hold a proper memorial service and belt out the hymns she so loved from her childhood.

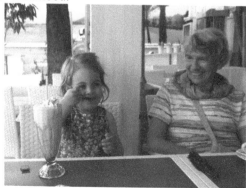

E and Dorothy (Mamgu)

I would always do some weeding or pruning in her garden, for which she was very grateful, being unable to do it herself. The combination of her punishing rheumatoid arthritis, rendering her joints weak and painful, plus poor lung function from the emphysema, reduced her to an invalid. E used to help me sometimes, but really, she just wanted to pop open her mamgu's* fuchsia buds. When my brother-in-law moved in to help care for her, he brought with him a group of cheerful gnomes, which amused me as I pottered around them.

Welsh for grandmother, pronounced mam-gee

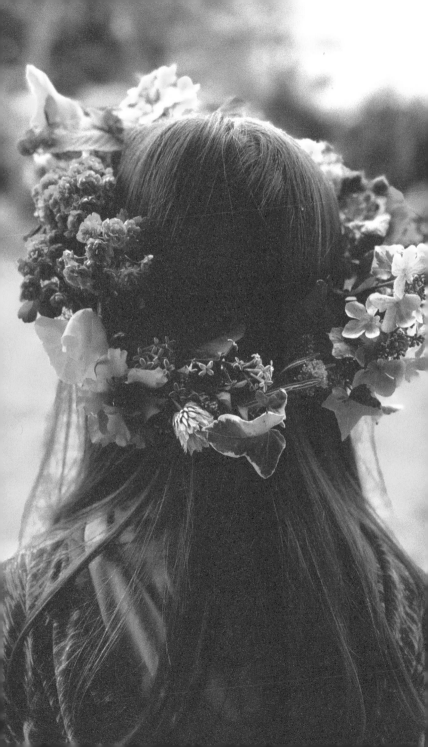

Chapter 26

I 've had a medium-sized garden for nearly ten years now. With careful consideration and some happy accidents, I have ensured that we've been regularly wowed by small wonders of nature. I embrace nostalgia by planting things I remember from my childhood or associate with someone I love. When I see or smell strawberries or tomatoes, I feel a warm glow and am back to eating them as a child, warmed by the August sun. Mum and Dad always had a small greenhouse in their garden, and I loved nothing better than sliding open the rickety door to breathe in the air, feeling a million miles away from the world outside. The smell is all at once sweet and spicy, earthy and piquant.

I've been growing pretty flowers to cut and bring inside; it's also lovely to pick them for other people. This year, alongside my vegetables, I will be growing gladioli, dahlia and cosmos, old favourites popular once more, driven by pretty pictures on social media. I choose bulbs because they require less water and cosmos because they keep flowering for weeks.

Grasses are sited to get the first or last of the day's low sunshine, inspired by a gravel grass garden in Mum and

Dad's Suffolk house. The graceful seed heads create stunning shadows, and I'm constantly looking at them and taking photos. They emerge much later than other plants, so it's even more of a thrill when they materialise.

Repetition is very pleasing. I try and plant in trios at a minimum, or more if I have room. Circular shapes pepper the back garden, including clipped pittosporum and box balls and gently swaying alliums, which sit atop long, tall stems.

I am on a never-ending mission to create a year-round garden. If you only buy plants once a year, the other three seasons will look sad in comparison. Each month I relook at the image in front of me and endeavour to fill the gaps, cherishing plants that happily grow through each other or that have different, complementary growth habits.

Winter reveals the garden's structure, and it's when I brighten up sparser months by filling old-fashioned Yorkshire flowerpots with colourful and textural plants, placing them by windows and doors. As well as creating my own pleasure palace, I am also giving rise to a mini wildlife reserve. Bronze feathery fennel grows huge and, this winter, I've had blue tits and warblers feeding on the seeds.

Spring can be slow to emerge, so giant bumblebees give thanks for early sources of nectar, and there is nothing more joyful than seeing shoots coming up when the rest of the garden is still resting. This morning I noticed an iris had popped up after yesterday's warmer weather – 'Katharine Hodgkin' is pale blue with perfect dark blue and yellow markings. She only has two flowers, but against the bare earth it is enough to really make me smile.

Late spring into summer is a time of abundance, when the plants grow more than you think is possible, and I revel in the lushness which delights me anew each year. The leaves and lime green flowers of alchemilla mollis push up to hide bare stems at the bottom of my egg-yolk-yellow rose, which is yet to get going. There are flowers everywhere, and the insects are in their element.

Midsummer into autumn can be overlooked, but for me, it's when my grasses come into their own. Combined with salvia, sedum and long-flowering geraniums, they keep the floral festival going until the first frosts.

Is there anything more wonderful than watching a bird having a dip, bobbing its head and back into the water and shaking freely from head to tail? We have a birdbath nestled in the flower bed in the back garden, seen from our dining table. In the front is a barrel pond with a pebble beach, great for both birds and pollinating insects on those long, hot, arid days with no rain in sight.

Autumn starts to show the garden's shape again. Colours become more muted, and seed heads stand proud as they turn brown, becoming no less attractive. We've had redwings, fieldfares, mistle thrushes, song thrushes and blackbirds feeding on our neighbours' holly, cotoneaster and sorbus berries. Without the berries, we wouldn't see all of these birds and I'm now planting some on our side of the fence. We fill bird feeders with sunflower seeds to attract goldfinches and greenfinches. Every day I watch and smile. Today a sparrowhawk swooped past the kitchen window.

It's also worth paying extra attention to your garden when the weather or season changes. Heat, cold, snow or rain can change the behaviour of animals and birds and make them likely to be seen in different places or doing unusual things.

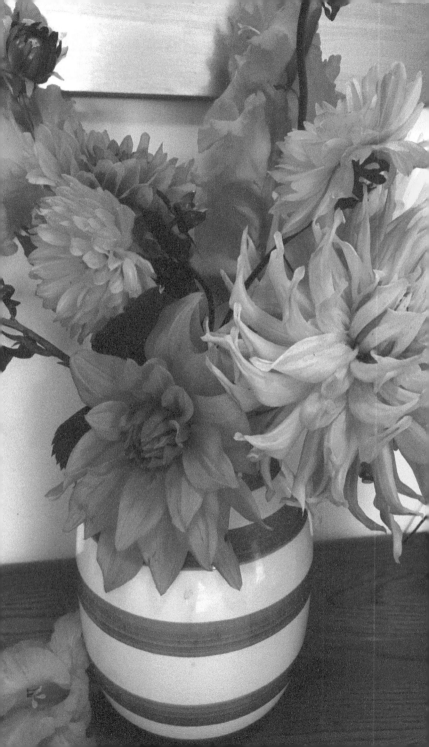

Epilogue

In a bid to improve my life – both with marginal health gains and more generally – I collect pieces of information like a magpie looking for shiny trinkets. Snippets from podcasts and radio shows, thoughts from conversations with friends, lines from many, many books; they all flow into me and some stick. I try to learn from them, to make changes, but there is a tidal wave of options.

I've tried so many things over the years. Not all have made a difference, but some really have, so my quest for better health continues. Just a teeny improvement here and there can all add up.

I try not to impress everything I learn on family, friends and colleagues, knowing they need to hear the right thing at the right time for them. Not everyone appreciates my forward momentum. Inevitably, much bubbles out. From childhood I have been a problem solver, a facilitator. I am still the little girl who wanted to make things better.

I'm thankful my past depression could be fixed with counselling and I doubt I would slip into it again - although life will have its own designs. I'm ultra-aware of signs that my mental health is on the decline, and if it is getting worse,

I tell someone how I feel, put myself first, and as author Katherine May portrays so beautifully, bring about a period of retreat or 'wintering'.

Strange things have stayed with me. I can find it hard to pick up the phone to friends. I still find goodbyes and endings difficult, making me unashamedly tearful. When I was depressed, I withdrew into myself. I'm an extrovert but even now I can still feel edgy before going out, although you wouldn't know it to see me. Even if I am with people I trust and love, I can get butterflies. The anxiety that crops up the most is whether I will have the energy to stay up. I worry I'll exhaust myself but, generally, once I'm out I get swept up in the buzz, and the worries drift away. I've learned to acknowledge the feeling but not let it stop me from doing anything.

My past experiences of illness and depression, and ongoing mild fatigue, continue to make me question anything that could adversely affect my health. Not drinking alcohol provides me with extra nervousness on a night out because I am no longer part of the exuberant drinking tribe. I don't want to feel left out, or for people to think I'm not any fun. But I hate hangovers, and I have no desire to feel rubbish and tired. The odd glass of sherry or port is about my limit now, or perhaps a glass of wine with a special meal. I remind myself that, once people get quite drunk, I am not missing much anyway and am better off home in bed.

I call myself recovered from FND, but in the process of writing this book I've wondered if I am. I've come far enough to be living a good life but my nervous system can still play up and I feel it keenly some days.

Today, my fingers are tingling, and I am very on edge. I am in the Stone Age forest, alert to every threat and ready to flee should the arrows come flying my way. I may be safe in my modern, centrally heated home, but my brain is prehistoric and doesn't realise that danger has passed. My bones ache like my skeleton has suddenly doubled in weight. Even my thin wrists seem like they are made of lead and, as I type these words, I am weary.

I can function, but it's not easy. My brain is in a foggy, spongy state, and my close-up vision is a bit more blurred than normal. I've learned to read quickly before things blur, but today even that doesn't help. The wrong words come out – spelling the word 'grow' out on a Zoom call, I say 'g-r-o-y'. I ask D if he wants a cold drink when I mean a hot one. I know what I want to say, but the signals are jumbled. I am chilly and sit with a microwavable heat pack around my neck. The warmth of each hot wheat kernel seeps in, but I am freezing again as soon as they cool down.

I feel like I could have a nap, but instead I potter around the garden and plant a few things. It's cold outside, but moving around warms me up and, after being productive for a bit, I feel much better.

I have always been restless like the wind, searching for somewhere new to land. I have piles of books on the go, spread around the house to dilute the true number. No one else knows I have signed up to five online courses in the last year and only completed one. I leave the hob to go and cram in another task, coming back to just-caught-in-time meals or sad, burnt offerings which are beyond rescue. Post-it notes and scraps of paper litter my desk at home. Ideas, tasks and thoughts spill out of me like a raging waterfall.

When I'm surrounded by flora and fauna, the impatient wind blows itself out. Adrenaline subsides. I am happy to walk and talk, stand and stare or simply sit and soak up the green, and just be. Being creative has a similar effect but I've learned I need to go along to sewing or art classes, or commit to doing things with other people, else even my best intentions never come to anything.

My IBS is an example of my brain sending the wrong signal to my body, in this case my stomach and digestive system. My symptoms typically flare up on days when I'm anxious, and the trapped wind can be painful. I'm lucky that, if I am having a bad morning, I can go to work a bit later without needing to provide an explanation. I am able to flex my job around any ailments, so I'm less defined by them. Treating it is a work in progress. I'm currently trialling a temporary FODMAP exclusion diet, followed by testing of different FODMAP foods to see which I react to, under the guidance of a dietician.

My IBS seems to be worse at certain times of the month. I've downloaded the Moody app, which tries to help women better understand their hormonal cycle and suggests natural support to bolster well-being. After reading the founder's book of the same name, I wanted to know more. It is liberating to think that I can better understand what's going on and be proactive in reducing symptoms such as irritability, water retention and abdominal pain. I've suffered all my life with period pains and related symptoms, and my health and energy always dip at the same time each month.

I've also downloaded the NERVA hypnotherapy app, specially designed to help people with IBS. So, typically, I am now trying more than one health solution, which makes it difficult to know if anything is helping. Am I scattergun or sensible?

Sometimes, in bed, I wake up sweating and stifled. It's only recently that I've wondered if some of my current symptoms, like brain fog, could now be the perimenopause rather than FND, so I've bought a book and am in the process of educating myself.

I have days when I'm not tired, but many when I am. Sometimes I soldier on, and other days I succumb to its grip and have a bath and an early night. I used to need regular daytime naps, but I can't remember the last one I had.

For a long time, I got cross with my body and grieved for all the things I couldn't do. Like running away from your shadow, you can never get away from chronic poor health. The list grew longer, and I grew sadder. I can't have a second child, work more hours, go on holiday to a scorching hot country, spend a whole day walking or climb Mount Snowdon. I know if I have more than one late night out in a week, catch a virus or have a busy time at work, I may suffer for it with a period of fatigue.

Now my mindset has changed and most of the time I don't define myself through my health. I focus on the many things I can still achieve, and am incredibly thankful that I've got better when not everyone with FND is so lucky. I've learnt that my health is not black and white. More often than not there hasn't been a magic fix and answers have to come from within, or from many different places.

This month, I've watched three episodes of an experimental online documentary designed to improve attitudes to uncertainty. It's been eye-opening, reminding me that my health challenges have given me a different perspective and made me a stronger person. Psychologists would call this post-traumatic growth. Popular culture regularly reminds us that what doesn't kill you makes you stronger.

In one of the episodes, a neuroscientist, Dr Vivienne Ming, told us to write down our greatest fear and take baby steps towards it, to walk into the deep end of our lives. What is my deep end?

I learn about our reticular activating system, a bundle of nerves in the brain which helps filter what goes into our conscious thought because the brain cannot possibly focus on, or remember, all the bits of information it receives in every second. We're told that humans can prime this system with active intention: to show it our dreams and aspirations and tell it to look for opportunities around the right things. So, by seeking out images for my one good picture a day, and intentionally noticing small wonders of nature, was I unknowingly retraining my brain to look away from the health issue of the day and towards something more positive? I have always known it worked, but it's interesting to hear some of the science behind it.

If I think about how much fitter I would like to be, my chest tightens and I can feel my heart beating like loud footsteps echoing over a wooden bridge. Instead, I focus on what's achievable and take small steps to keep pushing the boundaries. Movement is possible, even enjoyable. My tai chi teacher has since retired. I still complete the tai chi circles on days when I feel a bit twitchy or edgy, but I need to find a new class to turn an intention into a habit. Restorative yoga has been recommended but I am yet to find out more.

My weekly swimming, gardening and walking continues and I've come an awful long way since those daily London ambles when just putting one foot in front of the other was a challenge. Movement is a chance to zone out and connect with my body. Having done a mindfulness course, I can appreciate when I am in a mindful state and enjoy being there. Sometimes it can be as simple as purposely feeling the wooden handle of the spade in my hands, gazing up to find animals in the clouds or taking a moment to brush my fingers through rosemary, bringing them close to my nostrils and breathing deeply.

Last weekend, after I spent the morning feeling irritable and stressed, I moved two cubic metres of homemade mulch from the compost heap to the flower beds to counter the heavy clay soil. I must have been feeling physically good – it's not every day I'd have the energy to attempt this.

I shifted a lot of compost, but my negative thoughts stayed put. Whilst I had moments where the action of digging completely filled my mind, I kept circling back and then started catastrophising. I thought vividly about how things could get worse; the scenarios played out like watching TV. I've learned not to pay too much attention when this happens. I kept on moving compost until my limbs told me to stop. The pictures lingered; that day there was no easy fix, but I remained optimistic. These thoughts will improve, just not right now. Later, we went for a walk along the sea wall in Heybridge. The distraction of the river estuary and chatting to my brother and his family finally broke my cycle of negative thoughts.

I wake at 4 a.m. with a tickly throat and go downstairs to have a drink of water. Outside, a full moon known as the Flower Moon is disappearing behind my neighbour's greenhouse, orange yet hazy behind thin cloud. In some cultures, it's also known as the Corn Planting Moon or Milking Moon. This year, because it is a supermoon combined with a lunar eclipse that will be visible in some countries, it is called the Blood Moon and is bigger, brighter and more orange than usual.

Opening the back door to take a closer look, I am greeted by the dawn chorus, a non-stop, melodic sound coming from countless different birds sitting within all the surrounding trees and shrubs. As this rich, harmonious sound fills the air, I feel nostalgic for childhood camping trips. It's the beautiful, rousing noise you hear when under canvas in spring or summer months. A blackbird flies across the garden making loud chirps and the spell I am under is broken. It's time to go back to bed.

Bibliography

Books I've enjoyed, or have been influenced by.

Health & well-being

The Stress Solution by **Dr Chatterjee**. There is a podcast of the same name. Sound advice.

The Grief Survival Guide by **Jeff Brazier**. A book I have recommended to many people.

The Madness of Grief by **Richard Coles**. An honest and moving read about love, life, addiction, death and being left behind.

Sane New World: Taming the Mind. **Ruby Wax** writes brilliantly about tackling mental health.

The Upside of Stress by **Kelly McGonigal**. I really believe in the power of reframing negatives into positives. Four years after reading, much of this book has stayed with me.

Constellation: Reflections From Life by **Sinéad Gleeson**. Some of the best writing I have ever read about illness, motherhood and being a woman. Warning, it is not for the squeamish!

The Clever Guts Diet by **Michael Mosley**. I really rate Michael for his books and TV programmes.

Gut: The Inside Story of Our Body's Most Underrated Organ by **Giulia Enders**. Simply fascinating!

The Sober Diaries by **Clare Pooley**. Having drunk too much in my twenties and early thirties before stopping when I was ill, I can really relate to her experiences of not drinking.

FND Hope website and neurosymptoms.org/en_GB are the best sources of information for anyone who wants to know more about FND.

https://uncertaintyexperts.co.uk/ – I took part in the interactive online pilot; it will be interesting to see where it goes next.

Plants & nature

Last Chance to See by **Douglas Adams and Mark Carwardine**. I read this as a child, and it opened my mind to the wider world.

A Year of Living Simply and Thinking on my Feet by **Kate Humble**. I love how Kate makes time to walk and think, look and listen.

The Natural Health Service by **Isabel Hardman**. An excellent summary of how we can harness the power of nature to heal, combining personal experience with interviews and research.

Wintering: The Power of Rest and Retreat in Difficult Times by **Katherine May**. I could see myself in her writing, having had my own periods of 'wintering'.

The Well Gardened Mind by **Sue Stuart-Smith**. An inspiring overview of the remarkable effects of nature on health and well-being.

A Still Life: A Memoir by **Josie George**. Josie takes us into her world of chronic illness. She has helped me to appreciate my life by being more in the moment.

Rewild Yourself: 23 Spellbinding Ways to Make Nature More Visible by **Simon Barnes**. Don't wait for nature to come to you. Get out there and find it.

If you'd like more book recommendations, I am on GoodReads –

https://www.goodreads.com/user/show/54011841-hannah-powell

**

I took all the full-page photos - my small wonders - in East Anglia during the pandemic, with my mobile phone.

About the author

Hannah Powell (née Bourne) is Communications and HR Director for Perrywood Garden Centres, that she runs with her dad and two brothers. When she was six years old, she wanted to be a cactus surgeon.

Before coming back into the family business, she had a successful career in PR and marketing, running high-profile campaigns for clients including Barclaycard and Domino's Pizza. She was part of the team that launched Global Entrepreneurship Week, an annual campaign to encourage young people to set up businesses worldwide.

She now lives in North Essex with her husband, daughter and many plants.

www.thecactussurgeon.com